Medical Impairment, Disability Evaluation and Associated Medicolegal Issues

Editors

ROBERT D. RONDINELLI
MARJORIE ESKAY-AUERBACH

PHYSICAL MEDICINE AND REHABILITATION CLINICS OF NORTH AMERICA

www.pmr.theclinics.com

Consulting Editor
SANTOS F. MARTINEZ

August 2019 • Volume 30 • Number 3

ELSEVIER

1600 John F. Kennedy Boulevard • Suite 1800 • Philadelphia, Pennsylvania, 19103-2899

http://www.theclinics.com

**PHYSICAL MEDICINE AND REHABILITATION CLINICS OF NORTH AMERICA Volume 30, Number 3
August 2019 ISSN 1047-9651, ISBN 978-0-323-68212-1**

Editor: Lauren Boyle
Developmental Editor: Meredith Madeira

Reprints. For copies of 100 or more of articles in this publication, please contact the Commercial Reprints Department, Elsevier Inc., 360 Park Avenue South, New York, NY 10010-1710. Tel.: 212-633-3874; Fax: 212-633-3820; E-mail: reprints@elsevier.com.

Physical Medicine and Rehabilitation Clinics of North America (ISSN 1047-9651) is published quarterly by Elsevier Inc., 360 Park Avenue South, New York, NY 10010-1710. Months of issue are February, May, August, and November. Business and Editorial Offices: 1600 John F. Kennedy Blvd., Suite 1800, Philadelphia, PA 19103-2899. Customer Service Office: 3251 Riverport Lane, Maryland Heights, MO 63043. Periodicals postage paid at New York, NY and additional mailing offices. Subscription price per year is $304.00 (US individuals), $600.00 (US institutions), $100.00 (US students), $366.00 (Canadian individuals), $790.00 (Canadian institutions), $210.00 (Canadian students), $429.00 (foreign individuals), $790.00 (foreign institutions), and $210.00 (foreign students). Foreign air speed delivery is included in all *Clinics* subscription prices. All prices are subject to change without notice. **POSTMASTER:** Send address changes to *Physical Medicine and Rehabilitation Clinics of North America*, Customer Service Office: Elsevier Health Sciences Division, Subscription Customer Service, 3251 Riverport Lane, Maryland Heights, MO 63043. **Customer Service: 1-800-654-2452 (US). From outside of the United States, call 314-447-8871. Fax: 314-447-8029. E-mail: JournalsCustomerService-usa@elsevier.com (for print support); JournalsOnlineSupport-usa@elsevier.com (for online support).**

Physical Medicine and Rehabilitation Clinics of North America is indexed in *Excerpta Medica, MEDLINE/PubMed (Index Medicus), Cinahl,* and *Cumulative Index to Nursing and Allied Health Literature.*

Contributors

CONSULTING EDITOR

SANTOS F. MARTINEZ, MD, MS
Diplomate of the American Academy of Physical Medicine and Rehabilitation, Certificate of Added Qualification Sports Medicine, Assistant Professor, Department of Orthopaedics, Campbell Clinic Orthopaedics, University of Tennessee, Memphis, Tennessee, USA

EDITORS

ROBERT D. RONDINELLI, MD, PhD, FAAPMR
President and Owner, Pinnacle IME Services, LLC, Johnston, Iowa; Staff Physiatrist, UnityPoint Health, Des Moines, Iowa, USA

MARJORIE ESKAY-AUERBACH, MD, JD, FAAOS, FIAIME
SpineCare and Forensic Medicine, PLLC, Tucson, Arizona, USA

AUTHORS

SCOTT D. BENDER, PhD, ABPP-CN
Associate Professor and Board-Certified Clinical Neuropsychologist, Institute of Law, Psychiatry, and Public Policy, Department of Psychiatry and Neurobehavioral Science, University of Virginia Health System, Charlottesville, Virginia, USA

DIANE BRANDT, PT, PhD
Research Director, Social Security Advisory Board, Washington, DC, USA

CHRISTOPHER R. BRIGHAM, MD, MMS
President, Brigham and Associates, Inc., Hilton Head Island, South Carolina, USA

LEIGHTON CHAN, MD, MPH
Chief, Rehabilitation Medicine Department, Clinical Center, National Institutes of Health, Bethesda, Maryland, USA

STEPHEN L. DEMETER, MD, MPH
Henderson, Nevada, USA

MARJORIE ESKAY-AUERBACH, MD, JD, FAAOS, FIAIME
SpineCare and Forensic Medicine, PLLC, Tucson, Arizona, USA

RUSSELL GELFMAN, MD, MS, FACOEM, FAAPMR
Consultant, Physical Medicine and Rehabilitation, Mayo Clinic, Assistant Professor, Physical Medicine and Rehabilitation, Mayo Clinic College of Medicine and Science, Medical Director Mayo Clinic Work Rehabilitation, Rochester, Minnesota, USA

JAMES J. HILL III, MD, MPH, FACOEM
Medical Director, Occupational Health, The University of North Carolina at Chapel Hill, Associate Professor, Physical Medicine and Rehabilitation, University of North Carolina School of Medicine, Chapel Hill, North Carolina, USA

ALAN M. JETTE, PT, PhD
Professor and Dean Emeritus, Boston University Sargent College of Health and Rehabilitation Sciences, Professor of Rehabilitation Sciences, MGH Institute of Health Professions, Boston, Massachusetts, USA

RICHARD T. KATZ, MD
Professor of Clinical Neurology (PM&R), Washington University School of Medicine in St. Louis, St Louis, Missouri, USA; Fellow, American Board of Physical Medicine and Rehabilitation, Fellow, American Board of Independent Medical Examiners, Fellow, American Board of Electrodiagnostic Medicine, Section Editor, AMA Guides, 6th Edition

LEWIS KAZIS, ScD
Professor of Health Policy and Management, Director, Health Outcomes Unit and Center for the Assessment of Pharmaceutical Practices (CAPP) (Est. 2000), Boston University School of Public Health, Boston, Massachusetts, USA

LES KERTAY, PhD, ABPP
Dr Les Kertay & Associates, LLC, Ridgeside, Tennessee, USA

MICHEL LACERTE, MDCM, MSc, FRCPC, CCRC, DESS, CVRP(D)
Associate Professor, Department of Physical Medicine and Rehabilitation, Western University, London, Ontario, Canada

ELIZABETH MARFEO, PhD, MPH, OTR/L
Assistant Professor, Department of Occupational Therapy, Tufts University, Director, Health & Productive Aging Lab (HPAL), Medford, Massachusetts, USA

CHRISTINE McDONOUGH, PT, PhD
Assistant Professor of Physical Therapy, School of Health and Rehabilitation Sciences, University of Pittsburgh, Pittsburgh, Pennsylvania, USA

J. MARK MELHORN, MD, FAAOS, FACOEM, FASSH, FAAHS, FIAIME
Clinical Associate Professor, Department of Orthopaedics, University of Kansas School of Medicine - Wichita, The Hand Center, Wichita, Kansas, USA

PATRICIA A. MURPHY, PhD, MS, BA
Adjunct Faculty, Department of Women and Gender Studies, University of Toledo, Toledo, Ohio, USA

PENGSHENG NI, MD, MPH
Research Associate Professor, Department of Health Law, Policy and Management, BU School of Public Health, Boston, Massachusetts, USA

PAULETTE M. NIEWCZYK, MPH, PhD
Director of Research, Uniform Data System for Medical Rehabilitation, University at Buffalo, Associate Professor, Department of Health Promotion, Daemen College, Amherst, New York, USA

R. SAFFIN PARRISH-SAMS, JD
Managing Partner, Soldat & Parrish-Sams, PLC, West Des Moines, Iowa, USA; President, Iowa Association for Justice, Des Moines, Iowa, USA

ELIZABETH RASCH, PT, PhD
Staff Scientist and Chief, Epidemiology and Biostatistics Section, Rehabilitation Medicine Department, National Institutes of Health, Mark O. Hatfield Clinical Research Center, Bethesda, Maryland, USA

ROBERT D. RONDINELLI, MD, PhD, FAAPMR
President and Owner, Pinnacle IME Services, LLC, Johnston, Iowa; Staff Physiatrist, UnityPoint Health, Des Moines, Iowa, USA

E. RANDOLPH SOO HOO, MD, MPH, FACOEM
Medical Director, Medical Dimensions, Tucson, Arizona, USA

PIERRE J. VACHON, PhD, MPH, LLM, Esq
Principal, Life Expectancy Consulting, Sunnyvale, California, USA

NATHAN D. ZASLER, MD, DABPMR, FAAPMR, FACRM, BIM-C, FIAIME, DAIPM, CBIST
Founder, CEO, and CMO, Concussion Care Centre of Virginia, Ltd, Tree of Life Services, Inc, Professor, Affiliate, Department of Physical Medicine and Rehabilitation, Virginia Commonwealth University, Richmond, Virginia, USA; Associate Professor, Adjunct, Department of Physical Medicine and Rehabilitation, University of Virginia, Charlottesville, Virginia, USA; Vice-Chairperson, International Brain Injury Association, Alexandria, Virginia, USA

Contents

When health providers become involved in impairment evaluation, they inevitably encounter administrative systems that adjudicate disability determinations. Those determinations take place in varied systems, each with its own terminology and processes, which can lead to confusion and frustration. Understanding historical and administrative context reduces potential for iatrogenic harm due tocaused by needless disability. The key to better health outcomes for patients involved in disability benefit systems is to understand the health benefits of work, advocate for the best health interests of patients rather than for specific administrative outcomes, and to communicate clearly and objectively with both patients and benefit administrators.

Approximately 1 in 4 adults in the United States have a disability that affects major life activities. This article provides a brief historical perspective of disability determination, and revisits the conceptual foundation for understanding the current models of disablement and their general application to the major US disability systems and nuances thereof. The expectations placed on the physician-expert examiner and why the physiatrist is ideally equipped to function in this role are discussed. The article is intended to provide a heightened awareness of the medicolegal framework, potential pitfalls, and other ramifications of such undertakings.

Injured workers deal with many struggles while healing, forced on them by problems within the workers' compensation system itself. The physician's role is critical in mitigating complicating factors that have a negative impact on recovery. The workers' compensation system is meant as a safety net, guaranteeing prompt medical care; therefore, the applicable causation standard is lower than scientific probability. Physicians treating

based on a patient's functional level, obtained using the Functional Independence Measure. Inpatient BoC is a patient's projected resource utilization during a stay at an inpatient facility, assessed using the Northwick Park Dependency Scale. At the outpatient level, function and BoC can be assessed using the LIFEware System. Measuring and monitoring outcomes of all care result in reduced health care expenditures, more streamlined patient care, and improved quality of life for patients and families.

All editions of the American Medical Association (AMA) guides rate impairment based on static deviations from population or personal norms in addition to rating based on interferences in activities of daily living (ADLs). The burden of treatment compliance (BOTC) method of impairment rating was developed as a stand-alone model to help overcome difficulties when rating internal medicine conditions, when normative metrics may be lacking and impacts on ADLs are not readily determined. With the sixth edition of the AMA guides, the BOTC model has been adapted to provide alternative operational metrics for functional losses associated with these conditions.

This article discusses measuring quality of life (QOL) loss in litigation. Case examples are provided. The complexity challenge in QOL assessment is more easily addressed since the advent of computer adaptive testing, which is used by physicians and rehabilitationists in the administration of psychometric instruments to determine QOL loss. It is now possible to write algorithms to capture QOL data through text-mining. If QOL domains and their factors could be accessed through text-mining, it would make for an extraordinary opportunity for much needed doctoral level research in QOL issues for injured workers in workers' compensation programs.

Causation determination has become the gateway to treatment and reimbursement in workers' compensation and personal injury cases. The science of causation is constantly evolving, which is improving our understanding of individual physical thresholds, associated risk factors, and individual biopsychosocioeconomic factors. New laws place constantly changing legal thresholds for determining work-relatedness and proximate cause. The underlying foundation for fairness is quality science to support decisions made by the legal system to provide the injured worker the appropriate treatment to restore their function and decrease their functional impairment and/or assist in determining appropriate proximate cause in personal injury cases.

> Life expectancy expertise must comply with court-mandated evidentiary standards. A proper opinion should abide by 3 principles; it should be generated by a qualified expert who applies proper methods to appropriate facts. Several common mistakes can make opinions unsuitable for admission into testimony by straying from 1 or more of these 3 principles. Examining life expectancy opinions in light of these principles allows consumers of life expectancy expertise to evaluate the quality of the opinions proffered.

> This article provides an overview of validity assessment in persons with traumatic brain injury including evaluation caveats. Specific discussion is provided on post-concussive disorders, malingering, examination techniques to assess for validity, response bias, effort and non-organic/functional presentations. Examinee and examiner biases issues will also be explored. Discussion is also provided regarding judicial trends in limiting examiner scope of testing and/or testimony, and risk of liability when providing expert witness opinions on validity of examinee presentations. The hope is to encourage physiatrists to become more aware and skilled in validity assessment given its importance in differential diagnosis of impairment following traumatic brain injury.

> Medicolegal expert opinions can be the source of long and senseless acrimonious debates when they lack the necessary qualities to be considered good evidence. In contrast, quality medicolegal expert reports contribute significantly to the proper and prompt resolution of personal injury claims in civil litigation. To this end, expert physiatrists must develop the medicolegal mindset necessary to survive and thrive in the civil litigation arena. Medicolegal core competencies needed for this endeavor are identified and addressed for what is a lifelong learning project.

> Any physician who has authored an Independent Medical Evaluation or medical record review can and should anticipate being called as an expert witness (EW). Litigants rely on EW testimony in most civil cases. The most common areas in which EWs participate and provide opinions and testimony are workers' compensation, personal injury, and medical malpractice. This report will become part of the discovery process, the process by which a party to a lawsuit can obtain information from another party or other entities involved in the lawsuit.

The concepts associated with work disability are not identical to those associated with medical disability. In addition to a worker's medical condition, the resultant functional limitations, and loss of participation in society, the injured or ill worker must often navigate a complex administrative system that often seems adversarial. This process is made less adversarial with the willingness to participate of knowledgeable clinicians. This article informs the interested clinician in regard to the unique aspects of work disability, including the issues of work accommodations, restrictions, and fitness for duty; prolonged work disability; and other return-to-work considerations at maximum medical improvement.

The Independent Medical Examination (IME), as it is commonly referred to, is currently a mainstay of the medicolegal system. The IME is typically a one-time interview, physical examination, and supplemental record review performed by an impartial (ie, nontreating) physician at the request of a claimant's legal counsel or opposing defense attorney, in order to provide focused answers to a particular set of questions intended to help resolve a medicolegal dispute over the claimant's alleged work injury or personal injury claim. IME services provide opportunity for physicians to broaden and diversify their expertise and scope of practice.

Life care planning is a method of estimating future care costs for patients with catastrophic disabilities. The life care planner determines an annual budget for care, including further medical and rehabilitative interventions, durable medical goods, disposable medical goods and supplies, and recreational equipment. After determining an annual budget, the life care planner must use scientifically sound methods of determining the patient's life expectancy in order to create a lifetime budget.

PHYSICAL MEDICINE AND REHABILITATION CLINICS OF NORTH AMERICA

SERIES OF RELATED INTEREST

Orthopedic Clinics
Clinics in Sports Medicine

VISIT THE CLINICS ONLINE!
Access your subscription at:
www.theclinics.com

Foreword

Impairment and Society: Efforts and Consequences

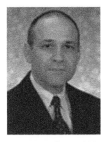

Santos F. Martinez, MD, MS
Consulting Editor

I would like to thank the guest editors for this excellent review. They not only deal with the challenging scenario of assessing medical impairment but also take us through the labyrinth of decision-making strategies, dealing with known and less obvious consequences. Disability in our society is reaching epidemic proportions, costing the taxpayer billions of dollars, much of which is attributed to musculoskeletal and neurologic conditions. It becomes paramount for our medical specialty to remain current in an effort to appropriately assess impairments and their subsequent impact on not only the individual but also our society. This issue certainly does not take the place of further concentrated study and coursework on the topic, but provides a very good foundation of information frequently not available. The authors and editors have vast experience in their clinical practices, including the inevitable medicolegal implications, and are active in national training efforts. I hope the reader gains new insights to enhance her or his acumen, addressing this segment of their medical practice.

Santos F. Martinez, MD, MS
American Academy of Physical Medicine
and Rehabilitation
Campbell Clinic Orthopaedics
Department of Orthopaedics
University of Tennessee
Memphis, TN 38104, USA

E-mail address:
smartinez@campbellclinic.com

Preface

Medical Impairment, Disability Evaluation, and Associated Medicolegal Issues

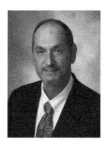 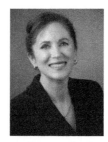

Robert D. Rondinelli, MD, PhD, FAAPMR   Marjorie Eskay-Auerbach, MD, JD, FAAOS, FIAIME

Editors

In 2001, I had the honor and pleasure of coediting an issue of the *Physical Medicine and Rehabilitation Clinics of North America* on the topic of Disability Evaluation.[1] My perspective and message to the reader at the time was that physician practitioners in the field of physical medicine and rehabilitation (PM&R) are ideally suited to embrace this area of medical practice because the essence of our specialty is the focus upon assessment and treatment of medical impairments, which arise out of illness or personal injury and have disabling consequences. Our training and experience involving functionally oriented goal planning and problem solving not only prepare us for the task of properly evaluating and treating the many musculoskeletal conditions that commonly give rise to disabilities but also enable us to maintain a realistic perspective on when the benefits of continuing treatment have been exhausted and, in cases of work injury recovery and personal injury claims, when timely closure at "maximal medical improvement" is both necessary and desirable.

In 2002, a separate issue of the *Physical Medicine and Rehabilitation Clinics of North America* followed on the topic of Medicolegal Issues,[2] including those typically associated with Workers' Compensation and personal injury claims.

For this issue, we have combined and revisited these topics with a selected focus on the collective efforts and shared perspectives gained through collaboration with colleagues from within and outside of the field of PM&R, and in particular, individuals who have contributed directly and creatively to the progressive changes embedded in the American Medical Association's most recent *Guides to the Evaluation of Permanent Impairment, 6th edition*.[3]

Phys Med Rehabil Clin N Am 30 (2019) xv–xvi
https://doi.org/10.1016/j.pmr.2019.05.001
1047-9651/19/© 2019 Published by Elsevier Inc.

pmr.theclinics.com

From both a conceptual and an applied standpoint, we have attempted to cover 4 areas of potential interest to help guide the physiatrist practitioner through this topic:

First, we have addressed the topic of impairment versus disability from 3 perspectives: the administrative viewpoint on these constructs as they are applied in the area of Workers' Compensation, and the constraints and expectations they place on the treating as well as the rating physician working in that system; the health care provider viewpoint as treating or rating physician; and the attorney's viewpoint when representing the interests and concerns of the patient as claimant in cases of compensable injury or illness.

Second, we have discussed the important issue of metrics for impairment and disability evaluation, including those traditionally available and applicable to the physiatrist (eg, impairment rating guides, functional capacity evaluations); and traditional and also innovative metrics for disability measurement, burden of care, burden of treatment compliance, and quality-of-life losses, which may, with further development or modification, become applicable tools to aid the physiatrist in quantifying disablement.

Third, we address forensic aspects of impairment and disability evaluation, including the topics of medicolegal causation analysis; life expectancy determination; symptom validation in cases of acquired brain injury and litigation; and medicolegal core competencies.

Finally, we address practical applications, including the physician acting as an expert witness; rehabilitating the injured worker to maximum medical improvement; the independent medical examination; and life care planning.

I am gratefully appreciative and personally indebted to all of the contributors to this issue who gave generously of their time and effort and, in particular, to my co-guest editor, Marjorie Eskay-Auerbach, MD, JD, for offering her incredible expertise, perspective, and insights in support of this project. It is our sincere hope that all of our colleagues who venture into the medicolegal arena of impairment rating and disability evaluation will find the issues touched upon in this issue to be at once stimulating, enlightening, and reassuring.

Robert D. Rondinelli, MD, PhD, FAAPMR
Pinnacle IME Services, LLC
6165 NW 86th Street, Suite 239
Regus – Foxboro Square
Johnston, IA 50131, USA

Marjorie Eskay-Auerbach, MD, JD, FAAOS, FIAIME
SpineCare & Forensic Medicine, PLLC
5610 East Grant Road
Tucson, AZ 85712, USA

E-mail addresses:
Robert.Rondinelli@unitypoint.org (R.D. Rondinelli)
meamd@mindspring.com (M. Eskay-Auerbach)

REFERENCES

1. Rondinelli RD, Katz RT. Disability evaluation. In: Kraft GH, editor. Phys Med Rehabil Clin N Am, 12(3) 2001.
2. Lacerte M. Medicolegal issues. In: Kraft GH, editor. Phys Med Rehabil Clin N Am, 13(2) 2002.
3. American Medical Association. Guides to the evaluation of permanent impairment. 6th issue. Chicago: American Medical Association; 2008.

Administrative Issues and Perspective: Impairment Ratings and Disability Determinations

Les Kertay, PhD, ABPP

KEYWORDS

- Disability determinations • Impairment • Benefit systems • Patient advocacy
- Work and health

KEY POINTS

- Impairment evaluations inform, but are not the same as, disability determinations. Impairment evaluations are medical; disability determinations are administrative.
- Understanding the historical context and language of disability benefit systems helps clarify the medical role, and reduces the likelihood of iatrogenic harm through needless disability.
- Advocating for a specific disability benefit determination blurs the medical role, and constitutes inappropriate advocacy.
- Work, and worklessness, have important health impacts. Focusing on work as a health behavior helps promote better outcomes.
- Clear communication of medical facts smooths the disability determination process and preserves the doctor-patient relationship.

INTRODUCTION

Disability determinations are 2-pronged: they require high-quality, evidence-informed medical evaluations of impairment, and they require accurate and appropriate application of legal, regulatory, and contractual language to determine whether compensation or other benefits are due to the patient, who is also a claimant and/or an injured worker. From the outset, this marriage of medical and legal systems is fraught with the possibility of misunderstanding, confusion, and frustration. This issue primarily focuses on making proper impairment evaluations, building state-of-the-art skill in applying medical science to impairment ratings, causation analysis, expert testimony,

Disclosure: The author has nothing to disclose.
Dr Les Kertay & Associates, LLC, 5 Crescent Park, Ridgeside, TN 37411, USA
E-mail address: les@drleskertay.com

Phys Med Rehabil Clin N Am 30 (2019) 499–509
https://doi.org/10.1016/j.pmr.2019.03.001   pmr.theclinics.com
1047-9651/19/© 2019 Elsevier Inc. All rights reserved.

and related issues that are primarily medical in nature. The first goal of this article is to forge a core understanding of the context in which those medical determinations will be applied. That is, to view the medical determination of impairment in the context of the disability benefit systems that will determine whether a particular medical impairment is compensable.

When disability benefit systems work as they are intended, patients[a] are materially supported during a time when they are unable to work in their usual occupations, or sometimes in any occupation, as a result of illness or injury that constitutes a medical impairment. The condition that causes the inability to work may be acute or chronic, short lived or extended, work related or not. Support is provided so that the patients can survive financially for as long as necessary until they recover enough to return to work, either to their own occupations or to another. Support is withdrawn when the patient can safely and effectively function, in life and, usually, at work.

Benefits are not normally intended to be permanent: support is provided while the patients are medically impaired to the point of work incapacity; they are helped to recover and return to productivity, and then support is withdrawn. This process sounds simple enough to be taken for granted. However, disability benefit systems do not always work as intended. Benefits sometimes are paid when they should not be, and sometimes are not paid when they should be. At times, the system breaks down and becomes an adversarial battle in which the patients, and perhaps their health care providers (HCPs)[b], feel obligated to prove their claims by exaggerating, or outright fabricating, symptoms and/or conditions.

From this author's perspective, there are 4 major primary reasons the systems sometimes fail. First is the failure to understand that, although impairment evaluations are a medical process, disability determinations are medically informed but primarily administrative. The second often follows from the first, and happens when the HCP advocates for a certain administrative outcome, rather than for what is in the best health interests of the patient. Third, HCPs often fail to appreciate the importance of function in general, and work in particular, as a critical health behavior. Fourth, HCPs may not understand how to communicate effectively with the other key stakeholders in the disability determination process, including, but not limited to, their patients.

DISABILITY SYSTEMS IN CONTEXT

One of the most frustrating aspects of disability benefit systems, from the HCP's perspective, is failing to understand the administrative nature of the process. HCPs are well trained in providing diagnosis and care, and can learn with relative comfort, if not necessarily ease, the process of impairment evaluation. However, evaluating impairment is a medical process; determining eligibility for disability benefits is not.

---

[a] In this introduction I use the term "patient" to label the person whose impairment is being determined. I also could have used "claimant," "injured worker," or any other description that might be more specific to a given benefit system. Using the term "patient" is both a convenience and an acknowledgment that these are individuals who are sick or injured, or perceive themselves to be. Whatever else they are experiencing, they are also in a health care system.

[b] "HCP" is used here to refer to the medical providers involved in evaluating impairment, whether as treating providers, evaluators, or forensic experts. In the present context, focused as it is on the evaluation of medical impairment, practically speaking that means mainly physicians, and secondarily psychologists and neuropsychologists.

The Historical Context

Offering care and compensation for individuals who become ill or injured is not new. As long ago as 2000 BC, the Law of Ur contained a scheme for compensating specific on-the-job injuries, and in 1750 BC the Code of Hammurabi offered a similar set of defined benefits. Many subsequent cultures developed their own laws that defined the ways in which specific functional losses (eg, the use of a hand, or the loss of an eye) were compensated. Central to all of these systems was that the benefits were an entitlement assured by being a member of society, and were offered when some illness or injury reduced the capacity to participate in societal life. By feudal times, these enlightened cultural codes were supplanted by the beneficence, or lack thereof, of the local lord, and, later, those of industrial owners and employers.[1,2]

Gradually, both public and private systems emerged to codify benefits systems, intending to protect both the individuals and their employers. The immediate precursor to modern private disability coverage began in 1848, when the Railway Passenger's Assurance Company of London sold the first accident insurance coverage as part of the cost of a railway ticket. That idea was imported to the United States in 1863 when James Batterson founded the Travelers Insurance Company and began selling policies that covered accidents during travel. Illness was covered, in addition to injury, when the St. Lawrence Life Association began issuing policies containing provisions for both. Thereafter, over time, policies waxed and waned in their popularity, benefits, and cost, influenced by both economic boons of industrial expansion and the busts of economic downturns. By 1956, Social Security Disability Insurance was added to the social protection safety net, in the form of a public disability program.[3-5] Central to all of these systems was the premise that coverage would be sought when needed (ie, when individuals were unfortunate enough to be unable to work), and only until they were back on their feet. However, there was also a cultural trend over time toward thinking of financial support as an entitlement.

Although private and public disability benefit systems focused on illness and injury without regard to whether it was occupationally related, the parallel development of modern workers' compensation systems focused exclusively on occupational injuries. Perhaps surprisingly, Otto von Bismarck was the initial champion of the precursor to modern workers' compensation. Driven by pragmatism rather than any great concern for the well-being of the worker, Bismarck co-opted the socialist agenda of protecting workers, and put in place the Employer's Liability Law in 1871. The subsequent development, in 1884, of workers' accident insurance codified many of the central features of current systems, including preferential treatment of injured workers on the one hand, and protecting employers by creating the so-called exclusive remedy that precluded other legal recourse.[1] This was the so-called grand bargain at the heart of workers' compensation: workers who are injured on the job are to be provided health care and income protection, but only for those injuries found causally related to work, and in exchange for which the workers gave up recourse for other means of compensation by lawsuit.

The historical context underscores several issues key to understanding how benefits systems work, and specifically the role of the HCP in them. First, there is an inherent tension between the provider of the benefit (the government agency, private insurer, or employer who is responsible for payments) and the patient/worker. The patients may be entitled to compensation by virtue of statute or contract, but only if they can show that their injury or illness meets certain definitions. Second, the definitions themselves vary over time, depending on cultural context (eg, become more or less sympathetic to the employee or the employer), the cost-benefit ratio (ie, the greater the likelihood of compensation, the higher the cost to administer the benefit; one way to reduce the financial exposure of the insurer is to tighten the definition of a compensable illness or injury), and the degree to which benefits are seen as a benefit or an entitlement (which varies over time and across individuals). In addition, and most important to the readers of this issue, at the center of these tensions is the HCP, who must balance the patient's health needs, the patient's desire for and (perhaps) sense of entitlement to compensation, and the demands of the system administrators who must ultimately decide whether to pay a claim, or not.

The Nature of Disability Benefits, and Their Language

The support provided by disability benefit systems can take multiple forms. The most obvious benefit is financial support, in the form of wage replacement while the patient is out of the workforce. However, there are other forms of support that can be equally meaningful. Providing physical and mental health care to help patients stay at work, paying for and/or directing care during workplace absence, financial assistance to pay for accommodations and/or assistive devices, and providing opportunities for retraining are some of the benefits that might be available.

Benefits are administered by multiple systems, each with its own sources of regulation and oversight. Public and private disability insurance, workers' compensation plans, and paid leave programs all provide various forms of wage replacement under different regulatory, contractual, and administrative definitions. Vocational rehabilitation programs, employee assistance programs, and other programs promoting both stay at work and return to work provide other material benefits. The systems and benefits overlap and are intertwined, but each has its own variation on language, definitions, and requirements.

A comprehensive description of all of the available benefits, across all of the systems that administer them, is beyond the scope of this article. What matters is that the HCPs should bear in mind that there are many different benefits available, each within different systems, each of which in turn operates under different rules and definitions. For a more complete discussion, readers may wish to consult Kertay and colleagues[5] (2016), Talmage and colleagues[6] (2011), and Warren[7] (2018). In the present context, some central definitions and concepts will help frame the issues that facilitate or impede the appropriate administration of disability benefit systems.

Impairment is a medical concept; disability is not

Impairment is a "significant deviation, loss, or loss of use of any body structure or function in an individual with a health condition, disorder, or disease."[8] Impairment is meant to be objectively measurable, and loss of function typically refers to changes in the ability to perform activities of daily living.

In contrast, although disability does have a medical meaning, in the context of the current discussion it is an administrative term. Different administrative contexts define disability in different ways. Under the Americans with Disabilities Act (ADA), disability is defined as a medical impairment that prevents the individual from performing an essential job function without an accommodation.[9] The important distinction is that the definition of disability under the ADA is designed to facilitate being able to work by providing appropriate accommodations. By contrast, the same word, disability, is used, in the context of public and private disability insurance, to describe the individual's inability to work. The same word, in different contexts, has a similar meaning but with opposite intent. [10]

In order to receive benefits, the applicant must be totally disabled under Social Security Administration (SSA) rules, which are influenced by age, previous occupational experience, and the physical demand level of previous work. Those same standards generally do not apply to private disability policies, which usually define disability differently, by contract. In workers' compensation systems, to receive income replacement payments, the injury or illness must also meet a standard of workplace causation, which is not required by other systems.

It is not necessary for HCPs to be experts in the myriad definitions of disability. The important thing is to recognize that a patient who is medically impaired may or may not be disabled under the relevant definition. Knowing that can help avoid confusion and frustration.

"Restrictions and limitations" is not a single, 8-syllable word

The key terms common to all benefit decisions are limitations and restrictions. These terms involve appropriate medical determinations of what the patient cannot do (a limitation), and what the patient should not do (a restriction). A more comprehensive understanding of these terms can be found in other sources.[2,10,11] Briefly, a limitation is a function that the patient cannot perform, regardless of motivation or tolerance. A fused elbow is a limitation because it cannot bend (lacks capacity). An elbow that has a normal range of motion but that hurts to move is not limited. Similarly, a restriction is a determination that it is medically necessary that the patient should not perform a particular function, because it is statistically likely to cause harm. Lifting above shoulder level immediately after surgery to repair a torn rotator cuff is a medically necessary activity restriction designed to prevent reinjury during an appropriate period of healing (the activity carries risk). Lifting above shoulder level later, after the initial healing and as the patient rebuilds strength, is not a medically necessary activity restriction simply because it causes temporary discomfort. If no tissue damage is occurring, the patient's tolerance may play into whether the patient wants to perform the activity, but that differs from a restriction.

Note that limitations and restrictions typically, but not inevitably, occur together. They are separate and distinct aspects of describing impairments in terms that can be applied to disability determinations. Using the torn rotator cuff example, a patient immediately after surgery is likely to be limited (unable to lift above shoulder level), and is also restricted because attempting to do so carries risk of doing damage. In contrast, patients with incompletely controlled seizures are fully functional (not limited) unless they are having a seizure. However, restrictions that protect the patient and others, such as restrictions from driving, working at heights, or working around moving machinery, are medically appropriate to reduce risk of harm.

In addition, it is important to recognize that restrictions and/or limitations apply to specific activities and capabilities, not broad categories. "No work" is neither a limitation nor a restriction, but a vocational determination. When claims managers determine whether the patient is disabled under the appropriate definition, they compare documented functional limitations and medically necessary activity restrictions to the requirements of the occupation. The task of the HCP is to provide the raw medical material from which that determination will follow.

Causation is a complex, specific, stepwise determination

The fact that a patient dropped and broke a phone in the doctor's office does not mean that the doctor's office caused the phone to break. Similarly, because a symptom occurs at work does not mean that work caused it. Also, because a car will not start after a rainstorm does not mean that the rain caused the car not to start. It might, or might not, have anything to do with moisture; that is a determination requiring specific expertise. Neither proximity nor temporal order are sufficient to determine causation, although they are elements of a comprehensive causation analysis.

Becoming adept at causation analysis goes well beyond the intent of this article, and readers are referred elsewhere for a more comprehensive discussion.[12–14] What matters here is that what seems intuitively obvious to the HCP and/or the patient may or may not be true. As with the definition of disability, determining causation is a medically informed, but largely administrative, process. Understanding that helps to reduce confusion and frustration.

PHYSICIAN ADVOCACY

HCPs often are, as a result of personal inclination reinforced by training, natural advocates for their patients. Ask most HCPs why they became a doctor, and somewhere near the top of the list is, most often, the desire to help patients. The problem is that sometimes HCPs forget to advocate for what the patient needs, and instead advocate for what they want, and/or think they deserve. When it comes to interfacing with disability benefit systems, it is easy to lose sight of the intended purpose of those systems: providing support while the individuals cannot work, and to stop providing it when they no longer need it.

Losing sight of this central concept is one of the key problems that leads to disability benefit systems not working as intended. HCPs are focused on caring for patients and evaluating their impairments; the defining characteristic is to provide whatever defines and promotes the patient's health. However, for administrators of disability benefit systems,[c] the issue is whether the medical impairment meets the contractual or regulatory definition of disability, such that benefits are due only for the time frame in which the definition of disability is satisfied. From the outset, having entered into an impairment evaluation, whether as a treating provider or an examiner, the HCP is in an awkward position. The HCP's primary concern is for the patient's health, but, once involved in a disability benefit system, the HCP is in a forensic role in which the health care and legal systems intersect.

The problem is that, in terms of patient advocacy, it is easy to see the relationship between claims, the physician, and the patient in adversarial terms. Benefits administrators have something that the patients want, and feel they deserve. Leaving out of consideration the outright malingering patients/claimants, who are a different problem altogether, it is reasonable to say that the patients come into the doctor's office, disability benefit system claim form in hand, believing that they are unable to work because of a medical condition. By initiating that interaction, the patients have placed the doctor-patient relationship at the nexus of a dilemma, and have complicated both the roles and the rules.

The patient is now both patient and claimant. The HCP is now both provider and evaluator. Both are now operating with a third party "in the room," namely the claims administrator. With or without an added case manager, the room can feel crowded with competing agendas.

If the patient has a measurable medical impairment, which the HCP can evaluate and document accurately, and the claims professional determines through vocational

---

[c] Typically, this is the claims professional (eg, case manager, claims adjuster, benefits specialist), embedded in a corporate or governmental entity that defines, administers, and delivers benefits to injured or ill workers.

analysis that the impairment precludes an important occupational function, then the disability benefit will likely be issued and conflict is at a minimum. However, there are several ways in which the interaction can go differently.

One problematic scenario involves patients who believe themselves to be impaired by conditions that, medically, are benign; for example, ill-defined low back pain without a demonstrable disorder and in the absence of any red flag symptoms. The patient has discomfort but has a full range of motion and no underlying disorder that will be harmed by being active. The HCP tells the patient that work restrictions are not required, and documents that fact, in which case a disability benefit will not be forthcoming. Often, a conflict then develops between the patient and the HCP. In this case, advocating for the patient's health involves telling the patient that it is in the patient's best interests and long-term health to remain as active as possible, including work.

If the patient becomes upset and demands that the HCP assign work restrictions, the HCP has a choice. Advocate for the patient's health based on what is known about benign low back pain, or write medical restrictions based on the patient's tolerance and what the patient wants. If the HCP chooses the latter, care is compromised, the benefit may or may not be forthcoming, and in any event the system shifts to one that is adversarial. If the HCP's opinion is questioned by the claims professional, or by a medical director associated with the claims payor, the HCP may decide to advocate harder for benefits, which is, in the author's opinion, the definition of inappropriate advocacy. Because of the nature of the system, the HCP ends up advocating for a position that is not supported by evidence, for a benefit that is not contractually payable, and that has no health benefit for the patient.

It can also happen that initial restrictions are appropriate but, as the patient recovers, become unnecessary before the patient feels ready to return to work. Patients may be anxious about returning, or anxious about reinjury, or simply may feel deconditioned to the ordinary stresses of work. Now, the HCP is in the same position at a different point in the cycle. Advocate for what is in the patient's best health interests, which is to return to function as quickly as possible, or advocate for a little more time to recover. Again, that extra time may seem harmless, but, as something that is not medically necessary, it represents inappropriate advocacy.

The motivations of the HCP at this point are not important, and in any case are complex. Financial incentives (fear of losing a patient), misunderstanding the nature of pain tolerance and mistaking it for disorder, animus toward the insurer, and pressure to move the patient along quickly and so failing to take the time to have a difficult discussion with the patient are all possible contributing factors. The motivations are rarely nefarious, but they nevertheless can contribute to iatrogenic disability and delayed recovery.

WORK MATTERS

At the root of most inappropriate HCP advocacy is a failure to understand the importance of work as a health behavior. Work is a source of financial support, a sense of meaning and purpose, and a critical source of social connection. Simply based on time spent, work is a central life activity. Working parents between the ages of 25 and 54 years spend more time on work-related activities (8.7 hours daily) than on anything else and more time than on all other waking activities combined. [15]

Work matters in terms of health as well. It is true that work stress is both universal and a source of potential health problems.[16–22] However, being out of work for any reason has negative health consequences that outweigh by far any possible negative effects of being at work. People out of work are more likely to be depressed,[23–25] to have heart attacks or strokes, and to die earlier considering all-cause mortality.[24,25] Simply living in an area that has high unemployment shortens life span, even after correcting for economic status.[26] However, those who return to work after a period of unemployment return to baseline levels of health risk, even when the individual dislikes the job. [9]

Worklessness, and needless disability, is also a huge economic burden. For example, the cost of chronic illness was estimated in 2005 to be about 10.7% of total labor costs in the United States. Most of that cost, 6.8% of total labor costs, was attributable to work impairment.[27] Lost productivity has an even bigger economic impact, with the cost of lost productivity estimated to be 2.3 times the cost of medical and pharmacy costs. [28]

Restricting a patient from work has significant health consequences. A useful analogy is to medication side effects. If an HCP were to prescribe a medication that shortened life span; caused depression; led to new medical comorbidities; negatively affected the patient's financial, social, and relationship status; and cost the patient enough that it had a meaningful negative impact on lifestyle, the HCP would recommend the medicine only after very careful consideration of the alternatives. The HCP would weigh the risk-benefit ratio, and have a long talk with the patient before going ahead. What would never be expected is to dash off a prescription for such a high-risk medication without carefully considering whether it was necessary, whether there were less toxic alternatives, and without documenting the rationale fully. Frequent follow-up would also be in order, including regular evaluation of the impact of the medication, including any adverse effects.

Understanding the real financial and health costs of being out of work makes the parallel obvious. However, in daily practice in the HCP's office, the same level of care often is not applied. To avoid inappropriate advocacy and the risk of iatrogenic injury, it is critical to understand the health implications of work.

ENGAGING WITH ADMINISTRATIVE SYSTEMS

Having explored the context in which disability determinations are made, and having described the importance of avoiding inappropriate advocacy and its potential to create iatrogenic injury, it is possible to offer some guidance to HCPs who are involved in impairment evaluations. What follows is advice for both evaluators and treaters, and is summarized from work that has been presented elsewhere.[2,11,29]

Decide Whether It Is in the Patient's Best Interest to Be Involved in the Disability Determination Process

This is the first step, often overlooked, especially by treating providers. Deciding to evaluate a patient for impairment, and assigning limitations and/or restrictions that certify disability, has an impact on the doctor-patient relationship. It complicates medical decision making by creating a dual role. On the one hand, the treating provider may be in the best position to understand the patient's history and to put the evaluation of impairment in context. The treating provider may also be in the best position to have a potentially difficult conversation with the patient, if the patient is medically ready to return to work, even if the patient thinks otherwise. In contrast, the treating provider may be reluctant to, and/or may be unable to, evaluate and discuss impairment (or lack of it) objectively. If the treating provider is unwilling or unprepared to be objective, the best option might be to refer the patient for a second opinion with a trained impairment evaluator, either through independent medical examination or a second opinion.

Support Conclusions with Clinical Evidence and Apply Evidence-Based Practice Whenever Possible

The need to do this applies for both treating HCPs and providers who are acting as independent evaluators. From an administrative standpoint, although the specifics may vary based on the particular system in which benefit decisions are being made, the medical professional is expected to provide clear, accurate, verifiable records and data that are thorough, descriptive, and legible. At a minimum, best practice involves 3 things: (1) establishing a clear and accurate diagnosis, based on recognized criteria; (2) determining the severity of the impairment, using criteria that are defined and explained in clinical notes and reports; and (3) assessing the functional impact of any medical impairment in terms of functional limitations and/or medically necessary activity restrictions. Understanding and applying the guidance in the remainder of this issue is a good place to start.

Communicate Clearly and Precisely

There are some simple rules that help maintain medical objectivity, reduce the risk of inappropriate advocacy, and promote the best health outcomes for patients:

1. Use terms that are relevant to the specific benefit system in which the determination is being made. Learn the systems, and ask if uncertain.
2. Use precise language. When applying a lifting restriction, for example, it is more helpful to assign a specific weight restriction than to say "No heavy lifting." Avoid restrictions that are impossible to follow, or measure, such as avoiding stress.
3. Only state facts that have been observed. If the patient reports sleeping badly, document it as a patient report ("The patient reported …"), rather than as a fact ("The patient sleeps poorly"), unless you have personally observed sleep.
4. Avoid speculating. Anything is possible, but possibilities cannot be used to make benefit determinations. Focus on what is more probably than not (ie, on the standard of medical certainty).
5. Let facts speak for themselves. Direct observation ("The patient grimaced when abducting the arm, but showed full range of motion") is more helpful than an embellished description ("The patient was in extreme pain when the arm was abducted").

Focus on Return to Work

Focus on, and encourage, return to work as early as medically reasonable and look for accommodations that will promote early, and successful, return to work. By understanding the role of the HCP in the process of disability determination, and staying focused on the potential harm that follows from unnecessary worklessness, the HCP can avoid inappropriate advocacy and promote the best possible health outcomes.

SUMMARY

HCP involvement in impairment evaluation inevitably leads to involvement in administrative systems that adjudicate disability determinations. The processes differ, but are entangled. Understanding the context, frameworks, and language of the system in which the HCP is working help to avoid the pitfalls of inappropriate advocacy and its associated poor outcomes.

REFERENCES

1. Guyton G. A brief history of workers' compensation. Iowa Orthop J 1999;19: 106–10.
2. Kertay L. Managing behavioral health in private disability insurance. In: Warren P, editor. Handbook of behavioral health disability management. Cham (Switzerland): Springer; 2018. p. 351–85.
3. Lynch K. Essentials of disability income insurance. 3rd edition. Bryn Mar (PA): American College Press; 2011.
4. Berkowitz E. Statement before the subcommittee on social security in Committee of Ways and Means 2000. Available at: www.ssa.gov/history/edberkdib.html. accessed August 15, 2018.
5. Kertay L, Eskay-Aurbach M, Hyman MH. AMA guides to navigating disability benefit systems. Chicago: American Medical Association; 2016.
6. Talmage JB, Melhorn JM, Hyman MH. AMA guides to the evaluation of work ability and return to work. Chicago: American Medical Association; 2011.
7. Warren P. Handbook of behavioral health disability management. Cham (Switzerland): Springer; 2018.
8. Association, A.M., Guides to the evaluation of permanent impairment. 6th edition. Chicago: American Medical Association; 2009.
9. Waddell G, Burton AK. Is work good for your health and well-being? London: TSO; 2006.
10. Kertay L. The health care professional's role in disabilty benefit systems. In: Kertay L, Eskay-Aurbach M, Hyman MH, editors. AMA guides to navigating disability benefit systems. Chicago: American Medical Association; 2016. p. 7–22.
11. Kertay L. Disability determinations and return to work. In: Talmage JB, Melhorn JM, Hyman MH, editors. AMA guides to the evaluation of workability and return to work. Chicago: American Medical Association; 2011. p. 115–33.
12. Melhorn JM, Talmage JB, Ackerman WE, et al. AMA guides to the evaluation of disease and injury causation. Chicago: American Medical Association; 2014.
13. Hyman MH, Kertay L. Causation. In: Kertay L, Eskay-Aurbach M, Hyman MH, editors. AMA guides to navigating disability benefit systems. Chicago: American Medical Association; 2016. p. 39–54.
14. Melhorn JM, Hegman KT, Genovese E. Evidence-based medicine and causal analysis. In: Talmage JB, Melhorn JM, Hyman MH, editors. AMA guides to the evaluation of work ability and return to work. Chicago: American Medical Association; 2011. p. 69–86.
15. Bureau of Labor Statistics. American time use survey - 2013 results. Available at: www.bls.gov/news.release/archives/atus_06182014.pdf. Accessed August 15, 2018.
16. Hauck A, Flintrop J, Brun E, et al. The impact of work-related psychosocial stressors on the onset of musculoskeletal disorders in specific body regions: a review and meta-analysis of 54 longitudinal studies. Work Stress 2011;25:243–6.
17. Kuper HM, Marmot M. Job strain, job demands, decision latitude, and risk of coronary heart disease within the Whitehall II study. J Epidemiol Community Health 2003;57:147–53.
18. Michie S, Williams S. Reducing work related psychological ill health and sickness absence: a systematic literature review [review]. Occup Environ Med 2003;60(1): 3–9.

19. Faragher EB, Cass M, Cooper CL. The relationship between job satisfaction and health: a meta-analysis. Occup Environ Med 2005;62:105–12.
20. Ford MT, Cerasoli CP, Higgins JA, et al. Relationships between psychological, physical, and behavioural health and work performance: a review and meta-analysis. Work Stress 2011;25(3):185–204.
21. Griffin MA, Clarke S. Stress and well-being at work. In: Zedeck S, editor. APA handbook of industrial and organizational psychology. Maintaining, expanding, and contracting the organization, vol. 3. Washington, DC: American Psychological Association; 2011. p. 359–97.
22. Donald I, Taylor P, Johnson S, et al. Work environments, stress, and productivity: an examination using ASSET. Int J Stress Manag 2005;12(4):409–23.
23. Psychiatrists, R.C.o., Employment opportunities and psychiatric disability. London: Council Report CR111.; 2001.
24. Thomas T, Secker J, Grove B. Job retention and mental health: a review of the literature. London: King's College London; 2002.
25. Seymour L, Grove B. Workplace interventions for people with common mental health problems: evidence review and recommendations. London: British Occupational Health Research Foundation; 2005.
26. Laditka JN, Laditka SB. Unemployment, disability and life expectancy in the United States: A life course study. Disabil Health J 2016;9(1):46–53.
27. Collins JJ, Baase CM, Sharda CE, et al. The assessment of chronic health conditions on work performance, absence, and total economic impact for employers. J Occup Environ Med 2005;47(6):547–57.
28. Loeppke R, Taitel M, Haufle V, et al. Health and productivity as a business strategy: a multi-employer study. J Occup Environ Med 2009;51(4):411–28.
29. Kertay L. Communicating with patients, employers, and insurers. In: Kertay L, Eskay-Aurbach M, Hyman MH, editors. AMA guides to navigating disability benefit systems. Chicago: American Medical Association; 2016. p. 55–69.

Healthcare Provider Issues and Perspective

Impairment Ratings and Disability Determinations

Robert D. Rondinelli, MD, PhD[a,b,*],
Marjorie Eskay-Auerbach, MD, JD[c]

KEYWORDS

- Biopsychosocial model of disability • International Classification of Functioning
- Disabilities and Health (ICF) • IOM Model: disabling consequences of illness or injury
- Expert witness legal considerations • Disability rating ethical considerations

KEY POINTS

- Physicians engaging in evaluating and rating disability after compensable injury or illness must maintain simultaneous commitments to the well-being of each patient and to the objective assessment of impairment to facilitate a fair administrative determination of disability.
- Delayed recovery after compensable injury is seen in a minority of cases but can have significant consequences in terms of prolonged and ineffective treatment and excessive costs of care.
- The ICF conceptual platform for identifying the disabling consequences of an impairment is an important tool for properly understanding the modifying influence (positively or negatively) of environmental and personal factors in the individual case.
- Physicians performing independent medical examinations and giving expert witness testimony should be aware of the additional liabilities associated with these activities.
- The physician examiner must confront the ethical challenges posed by an injured worker or applicant for Social Security Disability. This includes recognizing the need for objectivity rather than advocacy as an examiner when a referring party's interests and agenda may conflict with those of the examinee and their opposing counsel.

[a] Pinnacle IME Services, LLC, 6165 NW 86th Street, Suite 239, Regus – Foxboro Square, Johnston, IA 50131, USA; [b] UnityPoint Health, Des Moines, IA, USA; [c] SpineCare & Forensic Medicine, PLLC, 5610 East Grant Road, Tucson, AZ 85712, USA
* Corresponding author. Pinnacle IME Services, LLC.
E-mail addresses: rdrondmd@gmail.com; robert.rondinelli@unithypoint.org

Phys Med Rehabil Clin N Am 30 (2019) 511–522
https://doi.org/10.1016/j.pmr.2019.04.001   pmr.theclinics.com

INTRODUCTION

Physical Medicine and Rehabilitation (PM&R) is the branch of clinical medicine most dedicated to evaluating and treating the functional and disabling consequences of illness, injury, infirmity, or deformity that affects people's lives. According to recent estimates, approximately 1 in 4 adults in the United States (~61 million Americans) have a disability that affects major life activities,[1] and these numbers can be expected to increase during the coming decades. By 2030 an estimated 37 million aging "baby boomers" will be afflicted by multiple chronic conditions limiting their functionality.[2]

The medical field will continue to adapt to these changing demographics and the ensuing societal demands and expectations. Medicine will also capitalize on advances in medical and surgical technology, health awareness, and preventive care. Such change affords additional opportunities for PM&R physicians to participate in the formal assessment of impairment, resulting limitations, and the need for work or activity restrictions. The challenges posed by these activities can be effectively met by improved understanding of the conceptual foundation and terminology of disablement and application of same to the practices of impairment rating. By acquiring a rudimentary understanding of the rules and requirements of the medicolegal arena in which these practices are applied, the physician expert may facilitate administrative determinations of disability.

The purpose of this article is to provide the reader with a brief historical perspective of disability determination, and to revisit the conceptual foundation for understanding the current models of disablement and their general application to the major United States disability systems and nuances thereof. The expectations placed on the physician-expert examiner and why the physiatrist is ideally equipped to function in this role are discussed. The article is intended to provide a heightened awareness of the medico-legal framework, potential pitfalls, and other ramifications of such undertakings.

Although the words impairment and disability are frequently used interchangeably, they are not synonymous. For the purposes of further discussion, impairment is a medical term defined as "a loss, loss of use or derangement of any body part, organ system or organ function" and is determined by a physician. Disability is defined by the World Health Organization (WHO) as an umbrella term, covering impairments, activity limitations, and participation restrictions. In our current context with respect to any disability compensation system, disability is an administrative determination that takes into account medically defined impairment as one component. In this context, disability medicine refers to how system health care providers apply the science of ability, and disability, to all aspects of work-related or work-relevant conditions.

HISTORICAL EVIDENCE

Compassion for and tolerance of the disabled seems to be an elemental component of our social fabric, rooted in the very origins of human society. Many examples exist in the fossil record of earliest human societies whose members suffered and survived catastrophic injuries. The most impressive of these are the remains of an ancient human male excavated from Shanidar Cave in northeastern Iraq (approximately 60,000 years old) whose age at death has been estimated at between 35 and 50 years old. His cranial and postcranial remains clearly indicate that he survived a crushing blow to his skull that enucleated his left eye and resulted in right hemiplegia and atrophy of his right upper limb, which eventually autoamputated above his elbow.[3] Other excavations from a "stone age" site in southern Italy (~10,000 years old) provide compelling evidence that individuals potentially handicapped by dwarfism in a hunter-gatherer society were accepted and supported despite their nontraumatic physical disadvantage.[4]

There has been a long-held expectation that members of our human society must contribute individually to the common good to share its benefits collectively. It seems equally true that individuals who cannot contribute fully by virtue of impairment and/or resulting disability (administratively determined) should be afforded exemption from this expectation. In some cases, this compassion is exploited by individuals who engage in unfair or exaggerated claims of disablement. Our system of social justice must simultaneously compensate for bodily injury and illness and protect itself against payment of benefits to those individuals who avoid productivity.

Our systems of impairment, disability, and compensation have rules defining disability and entitlement as well as procedures outside the medical arena for determining who qualifies as disabled. These rules are designed to provide fair and equitable distribution of the system's limited resources to those whose needs are greatest and disabilities most compelling.[5]

CONTEXTUAL FRAMEWORK OF COMPENSABLE INJURY

As discussed elsewhere in this article, there is an ever increasing need for cost containment among providers working in the workers' compensation and personal injury claims arenas, and a few statistics readily underscore this point. Approximately 60% of annualized costs for occupational low back pain are directly attributable to disability payments, including lost wage replacement and indemnification at case closure.[6–8] Furthermore, a minority of the cases accounts for the majority of these costs (estimates indicate that 25% of cases account for 90% of costs) and 10% of cases exceed 75% of these costs associated with occupational low back pain.[7]

These increased costs have prompted the development of treatment guidelines and implementation of treatment strategies. If adhered to, these are known to substantially reduce the number of surgical procedures, work time loss, and overall costs by at least 50%.[9]

Favorable recovery, measured by return to work, can be expected in most workplace-acquired musculoskeletal injuries. Approximately two-thirds of work-related low back pain cases are expected to return to work in 4 weeks. All but 5% to 10% of cases are expected to return to work by 3 months, even though recurrent back pain is common in this group.[10]

Delayed recovery refers to an unfavorable response to appropriate medical and rehabilitative care over an adequate time period following a compensable injury.[11] Enablers and confounders of functional recovery and early return to work in such cases are well known (**Table 1**)[11,12] and need to be considered by both treating physicians and independent medical examiners.[9] As the duration of time away from work increases, the probability that an injured worker will return to competitive employment following a back injury decreases (the probability decreases to <50% at 6 months and to 25% or less by 1 year after injury).[13,14]

TERMINOLOGY AND CONCEPTUALIZATION OF DISABLEMENT

During much of the nineteenth and twentieth centuries, disability was conceptualized in terms of the "Medical Model" whereby disease causation was linked to underlying disorder readily identifiable at a histologic and/or physiologic level, arising directly out of illness or trauma. The physician's charge to diagnose and treat disease was extended to the diagnosis and treatment of resulting impairment.[15,16] With the advent of the stethoscope, microscope, radiography, and other technology, the physician was armed with instruments of precision and objectivity with which to determine the severity of impairment (at an organ-system level). This model worked best for

Table 1 Enablers and confounders of recovery after compensable injury		
	Enablers	**Confounders**
Medical	Minimal pathology Timely and competent assessment	Severe pathology Treatment delay Prior history of injury/prolonged recovery Poor cardiovascular fitness Inadequate exercise Job functions not addressed

Occupational	Expeditious treatment
	Employer concern and
	   advocacy
	Flexible options for return
	   to work
		Causality dispute/delays in work
		   compensation
		Startup or treatment authorization
		Employer apathy or hostility
		Lack of modified duty options
		Return to work too soon or too late
		Low job satisfaction

Psychosocial	Strong work ethic Acute need for money Facilitating insurance coverage Job discrimination averted	Poor English proficiency Disabled spouse/significant other History of substance abuse Anger or blame Prior or ongoing litigation Conviction of disability

From Rondinelli RD, Robinson JP, Scheer SJ, Weinstein SM. Industrial rehabilitation medicine. 4. Strategies for disability management. Arch Phys Med Rehabil 78;S–22, 1997; with permission.

unambiguous disease entities whose pathology was well understood and whose treatment goals and therapeutic end points were generally well accepted.[17,18] Today's "Medical Model" still serves as a fundamental basis for Social Security Disability determinations and for physician rating schedules, which remain largely anatomically and diagnostically based.

A "Social Model" of disability arose out of the advocacy movement of the 1970s and 1980s. Society became more accountable for disability as the inability to accommodate the special needs of disabled individuals became apparent. Limitations were identified with respect to environmental access and availability of adaptive equipment and discrimination, prejudicial thinking, and other attitudinal barriers were recognized.[16] This movement engendered closer scrutiny, better documentation, and improved understanding of the role of societal barriers to functioning, and helped foster strategies and tactics to neutralize these barriers and to enable and empower disabled members of our society.[19]

A "Biopsychosocial Model" of disability[20] has now gained wide acceptance as the preferred model when conceptualizing disability. The biological component refers to physical and/or mental aspects of an individual with a given health condition; the psychological component recognizes personal beliefs, coping strategies, emotional, and other psychological factors that may impact on individual functioning; and the social component recognizes contextual, infrastructural and other environmental factors that may also affect the individual's functioning in any given case.[17,21]

FROM THE CLASSIFICATION OF CAUSES OF DEATH TO THE INTERNATIONAL STATISTICAL CLASSIFICATION OF DISEASES, INJURIES, AND CAUSES OF DEATH

The World Health Organization (WHO) has created an international classification system of diseases and of disablement whose origins can be traced directly to the publication of Bertillon's *Classification of Causes of Death (ICD)* (1893) and, subsequently, the *International Statistical Classification of Diseases, Injuries, and Causes of Death*.[22] By 1948 the WHO began leading this effort and ultimately created the *International Classification of Impairments, Disabilities, and Handicaps (ICIDH)*,[23] which is reproduced in simplified form as **Fig. 1**.

This system was an initial attempt to relate the pathology of a specific disease or trauma to the resulting impairment (physiologic consequences in terms of signs and symptoms of dysfunction at an organ-system level), disability (functional consequences of impairment in terms of abilities lost in one's personal sphere), and handicap (societal consequences, freedoms lost in terms of role fulfillment). The relationship lends itself to being depicted in a simplified linear fashion and implies unidirectional nature and causation. This model fails to adequately account for confounders of a personal and environmental nature. More recently, the ICIDH has been replaced by the *International Classification of Functioning, Disabilities, and Health (ICF)*,[24] reproduced in modified form in **Fig. 2**.

The ICF system more aptly displays the interactive (ie, nonlinear) relationships between the impairment that an individual afflicted with a particular health condition might face; the potential functional consequences of impairment with respect to that individual's personal and social sphere; and the contextual factors that may mitigate or amplify these consequences including environmental factors, personal experiences, and choices. By taking environmental and personal factors into account the ICF has adopted the biopsychosocial model of disablement discussed earlier. The components of disablement according to the ICF classification system include the following:

Body functions and body structures: physiologic functions and body parts, respectively

Activity: execution of a task or action by an individual (typically functioning within their own personal sphere)

Participation: involvement in a life situation (typically within one's social sphere)

Impairments: problems in body function or structure such as a significant deviation or loss

Activity limitations: difficulties that an individual may have in executing activities

Participation restrictions: problems that an individual may experience in involvement in life situations

The ICF offers a conceptual platform for identifying the disabling consequences of impairment to an individual with a health condition (disorder or disease) whereby the

Traditional ICIDH model *(WHO, 1980)*

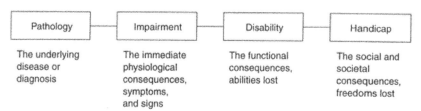

Fig. 1. WHO International Classification of Impairments, Disabilities, and Handicaps (ICIDH). (*From* Rondinelli RD, Duncan PW. The concepts of impairment and disability. In: Rondinelli RD and Katz RT (eds). Impairment rating and disability evaluation. Philadelphia; W.B. Saunders Company: 2000. pp. 17–33; with permission.)

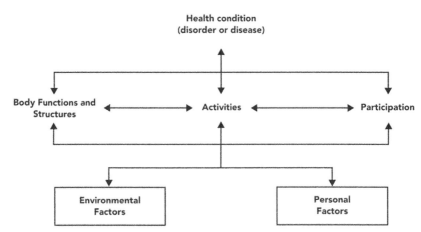

Fig. 2. WHO International Classification of Functioning, Disabilities, and Health (ICF).

modifying influence (in a positive or negative sense) of environmental and personal factors can also be recognized and more properly accounted for.

The ability to understand and apply the ICF conceptual framework is useful for both the treating physician and independent medical examiner (IME). In situations whereby an injured worker is not responding favorably to an appropriate treatment plan and delayed recovery is suspected, a critical review of environmental and personal factors can often reveal the enablers or confounders of recovery in any particular case.

By achieving such a contextual understanding, the treating physician can focus treatment strategies more effectively toward neutralizing the contextual barriers that may exist. An educated IME can consider the role of psychological and/or psychosocial confounders that may be operant. Understanding and accounting for psychosocial variables may be helpful for assessing the value of additional treatment intervention and recognizing when maximum medical improvement (MMI) has been achieved.

AMERICANS WITH DISABILITIES ACT AND IMPLICATIONS

With the passage of the Americans with Disabilities Act (ADA) in 1990, disabled Americans were guaranteed equal rights to employment opportunities, transportation, and public access. The ADA has its own key terminology and defines disability as a "physical or mental impairment that substantially limits one or more of the major life activities of such individual, a record of such impairment or being regarded as having such impairment."[25] Although broad and somewhat imprecise, this definition is narrowed under "Title 1" of the ADA (Employment) to recognize employment as a major life activity, and views disability within the context of performance of the *essential functions* of an employment position with or without *reasonable accommodation*. In 2008, the Americans with Disabilities Act Amendments Act[26] was signed into law effectively making it easier for individuals seeking protection under the ADA to claim a disability under the act, and made it even more important for the treating physician/disability physician examiner to understand accommodations and how important they are in the system.

Reasonable accommodation can include structural modifications of the work site to improve accessibility; availability of modified duty options; and acquisition of adaptive equipment or devices to enable an otherwise qualified worker with a disability to perform the essential functions of the job. Accommodations exempted under ADA include those that pose "undue hardship" to the employer in terms of cost or feasibility of implementation, or those that would pose a "direct threat" to the health and safety of the disabled individual and/or coworkers.[26]

As can be seen from the preceding ICF discussion, accommodation under the ADA is a social modifier mandated by statutes to mitigate the disabling consequences of impairment in the workplace as it relates to accessibility and participation restrictions. Most state workers' compensation systems do not have statutory language that requires an employer to take the injured worker back to work, and the employer may decide not to offer a return to work to the employee. Although the employer may be required to provide reasonable accommodation under federal statutes, the injured worker may no longer be an employee or, in the case of a small employer, the ADA may not be applicable.

The treating physician seeking to return an injured worker safely to the workplace is well served to review their formal job description and to tailor the ensuing therapy treatment plan to the specific material handling and activity requirements listed according to the essential functions. Return-to-work decisions can potentially be driven by the claimant's observed performance in therapy according to these essential functions. It is appropriate to return the individual to work when their physical performance meets or exceeds these requirements, or to offer restricted duty and to suggest accommodations when they do not.[9]

The employer is ultimately responsible for determining reasonable accommodation. It is not the responsibility of the evaluating physician to determine reasonableness of any accommodation proposed by the employer.[27] However, there may be value in the treating physician/disability physician examiner's suggestions for alternatives that would allow an individual with an impairment to return to work.

RELATING IMPAIRMENT TO DISABILITY AND COMPENSATION FORMULAS

Although the major current disability systems of the United States and elsewhere exhibit significant differences from each other, they all share a common mandate to compensate individuals financially for losses resulting from an impairment that also qualifies as a disability under regulation/contract.[28] The challenge becomes one of providing fair and equitable compensation for losses that typically can be expected to occur in 3 major domains: work ability, nonwork ability, and quality of life as depicted in **Fig. 3**.

An impairment rating provides an objective measure of the severity of loss of structure and function in terms of organ-system pathology. As such it is a key component of any administrative determination of disability in the worker's compensation system, although it may not adequately account for losses to the affected individual. Metrics exist to calculate losses to the impaired individual in terms of earning capacity, and these are commonly applied when actuarial analysis takes place. At present, there is no similar rating system for disability determinations under Social Security Administration or under private disability contracts.

In many states, the impairment rating becomes a surrogate for the disability rating. The American Medical Association Guides have gone to great lengths to distinguish between impairment and disability; however, current legislation and rules within workers' compensation do not necessarily abide by the distinction. The term "disability" is used in the administrative setting to capture the losses associated with an impairment determination. In such cases either a monetary value is assigned

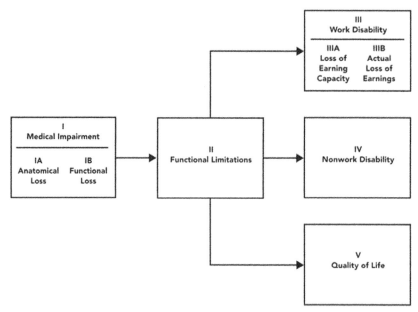

Fig. 3. Institute of Medicine: disabling consequences of illness or injury.

based on a statutory formula to generate a lump-sum payout, or a monthly payment is awarded to compensate for earnings lost, whether they reflect temporary or permanent disability benefits.

In summary, impairment rating is important to the categorization of disablement for several reasons:

1. It serves as a standard reference point in terms of linking a specific diagnosis to an associated percentage of physical and functional loss in compensable injury claims
2. It enables the impaired individual to exit the system of temporary disablement (eg, temporary total or permanent partial disablement under workers' compensation) at MMI
3. It provides a diagnosis-based classification of severity as a segue to alternative system management of long-term disablement[18]

The rating physician must be thoroughly familiar with the application of the rating manual or guidelines applicable to the case's specific jurisdiction.

LEGAL AND ETHICAL CONSIDERATIONS
Expert Witness Testimony

Physiatrists appear uniquely qualified among medical specialists to perform impairment ratings and evaluations used for disability determinations, because the scientific and medical foundation essential to PM&R is focused on human functioning. The knowledge, skills, and abilities of any physiatrist can be naturally extended to practicing within the emerging field of disability medicine. Disability medicine has been described as a subspecialty of clinical medicine encompassing the identification, prediction, prevention, assessment, evaluation, and management of impairment and disability, both in individuals and populations.[29] Expertise in this field extends to providing expert testimony in workers' compensation and personal injury claims in the medicolegal context.

The opinions set forth in the report documenting an independent medical examination are generally intended to clarify the extent of injury and/or impairment, associated physical limitations, and the need for work restrictions. This process is now a recognized part of the legal infrastructure associated with workers' compensation and personal injury claims.

The physician examiner should be thorough in gathering facts and available objective data. Opinions must be based on evidence rather than anecdotal experiences. The American judicial process is typically carried out in an adversarial arena where challenges to one's expert opinion are likely to arise. Opinions based on scientific evidence and sound judgment are, therefore, much more likely to withstand the adversarial scrutiny and challenge of even the most skilled cross-examiner.

Ethical Considerations

There is increasing ambiguity regarding the moral imperative of the traditional doctor-patient relationship in medicolegal cases. In the arena of workers' compensation the IME is at once accountable to the client (referral party) whose interests may conflict with those of the individual being examined, and/or with opposing counsel. In addition, the PM&R physician, by nature of his or her interdisciplinary approach, will consider maximizing functional recovery and reducing or eliminating dependency, to the fullest extent possible, on the treating system and caregivers, including the disability system itself. The injured worker or plaintiff is often represented by legal counsel, and may be coached and instructed, or otherwise choose to behave in a manner that is counterproductive to these goals and thereby appear noncompliant.

The physician must also remain cognizant of the paradox of compensable injury: that financial compensation can discourage return to work and thereby promote factors leading to an administrative assessment of disability. Undue prolongation of an open claim (through inappropriate and excessive diagnostic and/or therapeutic endeavors) may further serve to legitimize disability in the individual's mind, and can thereby reduce the likelihood of functional recovery and return to work. Decisions to terminate treatment of compensable injuries and to reach MMI may not always be mutually agreeable to the individual and examiner, and in most cases are likely to rest on the opinion of the physician.

Perhaps the most useful beacon to guide decision making when treating compensable injuries is to always promote functional recovery; to terminate treatment when functional recovery is no longer tenable; and to render impairment ratings and return-to-work decisions that enable injured workers to use their residual abilities (through accommodation if necessary) as soon as possible and to the fullest extent possible.[9]

The physician as IME steps outside his or her usual role as patient advocate. The physician's job in the context of an independent medical examination is to present objective scientific information. However, in such instances the physician faces the potential added risk of allegations of wrongdoing leveled by any disgruntled examinee who views the independent examining physician's opinion as adversarial to their claim. Serious allegations of financial,[30] physical,[31,32] or psychological injury[33] to patients in this context are a matter of record, and expert witness physicians are being held accountable if those injuries can be proved in a court of law.[34]

Until recently, medical malpractice actions against IMEs as expert witnesses failed because there was no defined doctor-patient relationship with the examinee.[35] Within the context of any IME, the contention was that the examining physician neither offered, nor intended, nor was authorized to actively treat the individual. Therefore, there was no established doctor-patient relationship to sustain a medical malpractice cause of action.[36,37] Case law from various jurisdictions has shifted to hold IMEs and expert witnesses accountable for the alleged harm suffered by the examinee.

At least two states' Supreme Courts have allowed civil action against IMEs to proceed under traditional medical malpractice theory in the past decade. The underlying cause of action in these cases was based on a duty of care to the patient (despite the absence of any formal doctor-patient relationship). The Arizona Supreme Court in *Ritchie v Krasner*[31] allowed a medical malpractice case to go forward despite the absence of a doctor-patient relationship by essentially stating that the court cannot envision any public benefit by not holding every doctor accountable to their duty to conform to the legal standard of reasonable care.

It should be emphasized that even though the recent case law in some jurisdictions has significantly removed the traditional malpractice immunity of providers who have no clearly defined doctor-patient relationship established with their examinees, considerable demand for expert medical witness services remains. Practitioners inclined to serve as IMEs are encouraged to attend several of the high-quality training programs offered in the United States to IMEs and expert witnesses, with the goal of empowering them with greater knowledge, skills, and abilities necessary to practice as an IME and/or expert witness in disability medicine.

In summary, physiatrists and other practitioners in disability medicine performing independent medical examinations and giving expert testimony should be aware of not only the legal liabilities in the overall practice of their subspecialty but also the additional malpractice and civil liabilities entailed with exposure to the practice constraints under which IMEs and expert witness work are performed.

IMEs and expert witnesses can be successful despite these challenges if they remember several key principles including intellectual honesty, professionalism, and respect of judicial process at all times. An ethical and objective examiner who performs a thorough evaluation, deals with the individual in an empathetic, unbiased manner, and avoids advocacy, has a lesser risk of becoming entangled in allegations of wrongdoing.

SUMMARY

Physicians engaged in evaluating and rating impairment and MMI after compensable injury or illness must remain aware of how this function differs from providing patient care. Delayed recovery after compensable injury is seen in a minority of cases but can have significant consequences in terms of prolonged and ineffective treatment and excessive costs of care. The ICF conceptual platform for identifying the disabling consequences of impairment can help the treating and/or disability examining physician to achieve a proper contextual understanding and facilitate recognition of significant environmental and personal barriers to recovery of function. Identifying enablers and confounders of functional recovery in such cases will assist the physician in achieving resolution of symptoms and functional loss to the fullest extent feasible; timely and appropriate determination of MMI; and deriving associated impairment ratings that enable fair and appropriate disability determinations at the organ-system level.

REFERENCES

1. CDC. Prevalence of disabilities and health care access by disability status and type among adults—United States, 2016. MMWR Morb Mortal Wkly Rep 2018; 67(32):882–7.

2. American Hospital Association; First Consulting Group. When I'm 64: how boomers will change health care. Chicago: American Hospital Association; 2007. p. 23.

3. Trinkhaus E, Zimmerman MR. Trauma among the Shanidar Neanderthals. Am J Phys Anthropol 1982;57:61–76.

4. Frayer DW, Horton WA, Macchiarelli R, et al. Dwarfism in an adolescent from the Italian late Upper Paleolithic. Nature 1987;330(6143):60–2.

5. Ranavaya MI, Rondinelli RD. The major U.S. disability and compensation systems: origins and historical overview. In: Rondinelli RD, Katz RT, editors. Impairment rating and disability evaluation. Philadelphia: W.B. Saunders Co; 2000. p. 3–16.

6. Leavitt SS, Johnston TL, Beyer RD. The process of recovery: patterns of industrial back injury. Part 1. Costs and other quantitative measures of effort. IMS Ind Med Surg 1971;40:7–14.

7. Andersson GBJ, Pope MH, Frymoyer JW, et al. Epidemiology and cost. In: Pope MH, Andersson GBJ, Frymoyer JW, et al, editors. Occupational low back pain; assessment, treatment and prevention. St Louis (MO): Mosby Year Book; 1991. p. 95–113.

8. Burton JF. Workers' compensation benefits and costs; significant developments in the early 1990s. In: Burton JF, Schmidle TP, editors. 1996 workers' compensation yearbook. Horsham (England): LRP Publication; 1995. p. 1–13.

9. Rondinelli RD, Robinson JP, Scheer SJ, et al. Industrial rehabilitation medicine. 4. Strategies for disability management. Arch Phys Med Rehabil 1997;78:S21–8.

10. Von Korf M. Studying the natural history of back pain. Spine 1994;19(18S): 2041S–6S.

11. Derebery VJ, Tullis WH. Delayed recovery in the patient with a work compensable injury. J Occup Med 1983;25:829–35.

12. Scheer SJ. The role of the physician in disability management. In: Shrey D, Lacerte M, editors. Principles and practices of disability management in industry. Winter park (CO): GR Press; 1995. p. 175–205.

13. Frymoyer JW, Andersson GBJ. Clinical classification. In: Pope MH, Andersson GBJ, Frymoyer JW, et al, editors. Occupational low back pain; assessment, treatment and prevention. St Louis (MO): Mosby Year Book; 1991. p. 48.

14. Waddell G. Epidemiology review: the epidemiology and cost of back pain. London: HMSO; 1994. p. 14–7.

15. Iezzoni LI, Freedman VA. Turning the disability tide: the importance of definitions. JAMA 2008;299:332–4.

16. Oliver M. Understanding disability. From theory to practice. New York: St. Martin's Press; 1996. p. 30–42.

17. Waddell G, Burton AK, Aylward M. A bio psychosocial model of sickness and disability. AMA Guides Newsletter; AMA Press; 2008.

18. Rondinelli RD. Changes for the new AMA Guides to impairment ratings, 6th edition: implications and applications for physician disability evaluations. PM R 2008;1(7):643–56.

19. Fougeyrollas P. Documenting environmental factors for preventing the handicap creation process: Quebec contributions relating to ICIDH and social participation of people with functional differences. Disabil Rehabil 1995;17:145–53.

20. Engle GL. The need for a new medical model: a challenge for biomedicine. Science 1977;196:129–36.

21. Waddell G, Burton AK. Concepts of rehabilitation for the management of common health problems. London: TSO (The Stationary Office); 2004.
22. World Health Organization. History of the development of the ICD. Available at: http://www.who.int/entity/classifications/icd/en/HistoryOfICD.pdf.
23. World Health Organization. International classification of impairments, disabilities and handicaps: a manual of classification relating to the consequences of disease. Geneva (Switzerland): World Health Organization; 1980.
24. World Health Organization. International classification of functioning, disability, and health (ICF). Geneva (Switzerland): World Health Organization; 2001.
25. Americans With Disabilities Act: Part 1. Employment (29 CFR part 1630). Federal Register, July 26, 1991, pp. 35726–35756.
26. Americans with Disabilities Act Amendments Act of 2008 – EEOC. Available at: http://www.eeoc.gov/laws/statutes/adaaa.cfm.
27. Johns RE Jr, Colledge AL, Holmes EB. Introduction to fitness for duty. In: Demeter SL, Andersson GB, editors. Disability evaluation2. St Louis (MO): Mosby/AMA; 2003. p. 709–38.
28. McGeary M, Ford M, McCutchen SR, et al, editors. IOM Committee on medical evaluation of veterans for disability compensation: a 21st century system for evaluating veterans for disability benefits. The rating schedule. Washington, DC: The National Academies Press; 2007.
29. Ranavaya MI. Presidential Address, American Academy of Disability Evaluating Physicians, 1997.
30. Greenberg v Perkins. 845 P.2d 530, 538 (Colo 1993).
31. Ritchie v Krasner, M.D., et al. 211 P.3d 1272 (Ariz. Ct. App. 2009).
32. Smith v Welch. 265 Kan. 881P.2d 727 (1998).
33. Harris v Kreutzer. 624 S.E. 2d 24, 27 (Va. 2006).
34. Rondinelli RD, Ranavaya MI. Practical aspects of impairment rating and disability determination. In: Cifu DX, editor. Braddom's physical medicine & rehabilitation. 5th edition. Philadelphia: Elsevier, Inc; 2016. p. 85–101.
35. Rand v Miller. 408 SE 2d 655 (WVa 1991).
36. Johnston v Sibley, 588 SW 2d 135 (Tex Civ App 1977).
37. Keene v Wiggins. 138 Cal Rep 3 (Cal App 1977).

Plaintiff Attorney's Issues and Perspective: The Injured Worker as Claimant

R. Saffin Parrish-Sams, JD

KEYWORDS

- Injured worker • Physician • Problems • Pressures • Bias • Causation • Disability

KEY POINTS

- Injured workers contend with many challenges while healing, forced on them by perceived and real problems within the workers' compensation system.
- The physician's role is critical in mitigating external complicating factors that can have a negative impact on recovery or prolong the process.
- The evaluating physician must recognize that legal causation differs from medical/scientific causation when opining on causation.
- Although physicians see individuals for disability evaluations or assessment, the determination of disability is a legal issue determined by a court.
- Disability evaluations are most useful when they thoroughly describe and quantify objectively manifested physiologic capabilities lost, added burdens, and subjective factors that could affect employability.

INTRODUCTION

In the workers' compensation system, the physician's role is both critical and pivotal. When physicians approach injured workers in the same manner as other patients, everyone in the system benefits. The injured worker who receives appropriate treatment most often returns to work and retains seniority. The employer regains a fully trained and satisfied employee, and, as a result, the insurance carrier pays fewer benefits.

If, on the other hand, the care provided is inadequate, everyone in the system suffers. Less than adequate care may occur when physicians try to please an employer or insurer who is focused on short-term gains, desiring to limit or deny liability, limit treatment costs, or promote a premature return to work. As a result, the injured worker may experience delays in treatment, prolonged or less than optimal recovery, reinjury, and other frustrations. The physician may be subject to the injured worker's frustration. The employer then will be without an employee for longer than necessary and is

Disclosure Statement: The author has nothing to disclose.
Soldat & Parrish-Sams, PLC, 3408 Woodland Avenue, Suite 302, West Des Moines, IA 50266, USA
E-mail address: saffinspslaw@outlook.com

Phys Med Rehabil Clin N Am 30 (2019) 523–532
https://doi.org/10.1016/j.pmr.2019.03.002
1047-9651/19/© 2019 Elsevier Inc. All rights reserved.

exposed to additional losses due to sequela injuries or conditions. Ultimately, the insurer is forced to set its reserves higher to accommodate the extended treatment, additional losses, and costs of defense.

Physicians involved in the workers' compensation system have multiple competing pressures—from employers, insurance carriers, case managers, the injured workers, attorneys, and physicians' own employers. In addition, an injured worker's rehabilitation may be impeded by complicated psychosocial issues and stresses related to the system itself. Nevertheless, a treating physician's legal, moral, and ethical duties to a patient do not change, simply because a patient was injured at work.

The no-fault workers compensation system was designed to be a safety net, ensuring that injured workers receive prompt medical care for injuries that "arise out of" their employment. Consequently, legal causation and medical causation are not interchangeable. Physicians, therefore, need to be aware of the proper legal standard when rendering their causation opinions.

Restrictions after recovery from an injury may be appropriate. Restrictions and functional limitations should be described completely and address both material handling and nonmaterial handling functions, such as activities of daily living, which have an impact on injured workers' lives. Fully describing the long-term impact of an injury enables the legal system to better assess disability and facilitates an injured worker's return to activities after an injury.

DISCUSSION
Injured People Are Human Beings, Not Trucks or Superheroes

Not all human beings have the same physical or psychological resilience. Human frailties and susceptibilities may predispose individuals to certain types of injuries or result in greater than expected disability from those injuries. In addition to physical factors, extrinsic and intrinsic psychosocial factors can play a role in the injured workers' response to injuries, pain, and functional loss. A positive physician-patient relationship, in the context of treating injured workers, may help an injured worker cope with and be motivated to overcome injuries, pain, and impairment. [1]

Unfortunately, too often injured workers are forced to deal with more complicated problems than just healing from the injury itself.[2–6] A 2015 Occupational Health and Safety Administration report found:

> The costs of workplace injuries are borne primarily by injured workers, their families, and taxpayer-supported components of the social safety net. Changes in state-based workers' compensation insurance programs have made it increasingly difficult for injured workers to receive the full benefits (including adequate wage replacement payments and coverage for medical expenses) to which they are entitled. Employers now provide only a small percentage (about 20%) of the overall financial cost of workplace injuries and illnesses through workers' compensation. This cost-shift has forced injured workers, their families and taxpayers to subsidize the vast majority of the lost income and medical care costs generated by these conditions.[7]

In my practice, as well as colleagues', the following are known to happen to injured workers:

- Injured workers often are treated with suspicion by employers, adjusters, and physicians. Their injury is questioned. Their motivation is questioned. Their integrity is questioned.[2(p16),8]

- Injured workers commonly report difficulty paying bills (eg, rent, mortgage, utilities, car payment, and groceries). Their temporary disability checks (wage replacement checks while recovering from an injury) are held up for weeks or months "pending further investigation," or are underpaid, or are not paid on time, or are not paid at all.
- Injured workers endure repeated and protracted treatment delays. Initial delays come from employers and adjusters investigating whether to accept an injury as compensable. Additional delays occur while waiting for the adjuster to preauthorize the recommended treatment or because a nurse case manager (NCM) changes appointments to fit the NCM's schedule.
- Injured workers report being told by physicians that they are receiving inferior or less extensive medical treatment because they were injured at work (eg, "I won't operate on injured workers, because studies show they don't have good outcomes"; "I would normally order X treatment, but work comp insurance won't pay for it"; or "I have only been authorized to treat your arm, and am not authorized to evaluate your neck to see if that is the source of the symptoms in your arm").
- In an employer choice state, injured workers often report that treating physicians are more responsive to NCMs, insurance adjusters, and defense attorneys than to the questions posed and treatment preferred by the injured patient.
- Injured workers are scrutinized or criticized for not returning to work or reaching maximum medical improvement within an expected number of days specified in a 1-size-fits-all disability manual. This occurs regardless of whether the carrier has delayed authorizing diagnostics, therapy, surgery, or other treatment.
- The nature, extent, existence, and persistence of an injured worker's pain, symptoms, and functional limitations are mistrusted or even dismissed, because of the unrelenting pressure on physicians to return them to work as soon as possible, by a for-profit insurance industry intent on cost containment.[9]

Some employers are accommodating and supportive of injured workers during their recovery. Some employers, supervisors, and even coworkers, however, place pressure on injured workers to exceed the medically imposed restrictions or to obtain a release to return to full duty work earlier than indicated (eg, imply their job is in danger; tell them to "man up"; complain they are slowing production and ruining "production bonuses"; or complain they are ruining the safety record and need to return to full duty so "safety bonuses" will be paid).

Sometimes employers cannot modify an injured worker's normal job to accommodate restrictions, and as an alternative, they place the patient in a make-work position. These positions can be legitimate, but can also be punitive (eg, scrubbing toilets and urinals and emptying feminine hygiene boxes, working in an unheated room, or assigning a single mother to a night shift when she has no child care) or pointless (eg, sitting in a designated room all day doing nothing or tearing the edges off dot-matrix computer paper).

These negative experiences can be frustrating and difficult, particularly for injured workers with less innate resiliency. Exceeding medical restrictions, returning to work too soon, and treatment delays may result in prolonged recovery time. These adversities can also lead to increased human distress, disturbed sleep, and further complications from mental health sequelae.

Consequently, by the time permanent impairment and disability are assessed, many injured workers have felt some degree of fear, frustration, pain, worry, abandonment, or mistreatment by an employer they believed they could trust. Thus, not all injured workers—with their unique human frailties, susceptibilities, resiliencies, and experience with the workers' compensation system—can be expected to have the exact same recovery outcome after a work injury. The optimal recovery, or expected outcome, when fixing a human injury is not as predictable or standardized as replacing a part in a truck.

The Physician's Role

Whether treating an injured worker, determining causation, or assessing impairment or disability factors after an injury, a physician's role is to be a physician. Although treating physicians should advocate for their patients, experts are expected to be independent and not advocate for a particular outcome in a case. Physicians must remain independent in exercising their best medical judgment.

A physician's role in treating injured workers may be complicated by several factors. Clinicians are under time pressures to see a certain number of patients each day: "Observers have noted that, on average, physicians interrupt patients within 18 seconds of when they begin telling their story."[10] Time pressures can negatively impact patient interaction when injured workers want to explain how they were injured and their symptom progression, and a case manager wants to use a portion of the allotted appointment time to have an employer's questions answered. In addition, the nature of the workers' compensation system can place significant competing demands on a treating physician: the employer, adjuster, and case manager want one thing, the injured patient wants something different, and the physician is in the middle.

Regardless of the pressures, treating physicians have legal, moral, and ethical duties to their patients. This is true regardless of the entity responsible for paying the bills. Therefore, treatment recommendations should be appropriate for the medical condition and not be based on what treatment a workers' compensation insurer may or may not be willing to pay for.[3(pp2, 4)] Physicians are expected to recommend appropriate and medically necessary treatment of the work-related condition. Whether or not an injured worker then receives the suggested treatment is a separate function of the applicable law.

It is incumbent on the treating physician to advise an injured worker of all medically reasonable differential diagnoses, treatment options, and associated risks, so that the injured worker can make informed decisions about treatment. Physicians should document all reported symptoms and reasonable alternative etiologies for those symptoms, even when doing so extends beyond the body part they have been authorized to treat. Physicians should discuss treatment options with an injured worker, such as surgery, if they would present that same treatment option to a patient who suffered a similar injury at home.

When a patient is returned to work after an injury, it is important for physicians to provide all medically appropriate restrictions. It is then up to the employer and injured worker to determine whether the employer can reasonably accommodate all medical restrictions or if the injured worker should remain off work. It is helpful for a physician to understand both the job description and the actual tasks the injured worker is asked to perform. It is likewise helpful to obtain the injured workers' personal experience in performing that job, so as to identify and make recommendations to neutralize any physical or psychosocial obstacles to recovery.

Medical restrictions should not be based on the availability of work. It is not appropriate to release an injured worker to full duty with no restrictions, simply because they have been terminated by their employer and have no job, or because they have a sedentary job that does not require prolonged standing or heavy lifting. An injured worker requires documentation of any medically appropriate restrictions related to the injury, because those restrictions affect their vocational and avocational activities, search for appropriate new employment, entitlement to temporary benefits, and legal assessment of disability. Some employers accommodate restrictions only long enough to get a case settled, after which the injured worker is laid off, or let go. When assessing permanent restrictions, physicians should list all functional limitations that apply in a generic work environment are important, rather than just current job-specific tasks.

When evaluating or treating injured workers, some physicians may have conscious or unconscious biases. The expression of these biases may be subtle or overt, but either way it is likely perceived by the patient.[1,8] When evaluating or treating injured workers, physicians should give them the benefit of the doubt, until given a good medical reason to do otherwise. A physician-patient relationship that lacks trust creates added distress for the injured worker, and in turn, complicates recovery.[1] Patients do not choose to be injured on the job or to participate in a workers' compensation system plagued by inadequate benefits and increasing hurdles[8] to obtaining medical care:

> Recent years have seen significant changes to workers' compensation laws, procedures, and policies in numerous states, which have limited benefits, reduced the likelihood of successful application for workers' compensation, and/or discouraged injured workers from applying for benefits. These include changes that have resulted in the denial of claims that were previously compensated, a decrease in the adequacy of cash benefits to those awarded compensation, imposition of restrictions regarding the medical care provided injured workers, and the institution of new procedural and evidentiary rules that create barriers for injured workers who filed claims… All these issues result in the transfer of the economic cost of occupationally caused or aggravated injuries and illnesses to families, communities, and other benefit programs, further burdening the federal Medicare and Social Security disability insurance programs.[2(pp2–3)]

Finally, physicians providing causation opinions, impairment ratings, and disability evaluations should base these opinions on the objective findings documented in medical records and diagnostic testing, physical examination findings of the patient, and medical principles and methodologies. An independent medical examiner should be aware of the risks of attribution bias and confirmation bias in performing their assessments. The American Psychiatric Association cautions that "assessment of conscious intention is unreliable."[11] Expert medical opinions are intended to educate the court, and there is no place for comments implying a conscious intent to lie or exaggerate by the injured person while ignoring other human factors[12] or psychosocial considerations that may affect the way an individual presents on examination, such as:

- Not all human beings respond to injuries, pain, and lost function the same way
- The effect of delayed treatment
- The effect of an inadequate family/social/employment support network during recovery
- The aggregate effect of attempting to communicate very real symptoms and difficulties to nonempathetic listeners
- The effects of pain (injured workers having no greater ability to present objective proof that they are experiencing pain than a patient who was injured at home)
- The effects of poor sleep (due to pain and anxiety)
- The effects of depression or anxiety (due to exacerbation of a preexisting mental health condition or as a response to the difficulties posed by the work comp system)

- The effects of medication (many have known side effects that interfere with cognition and function)
- Cultural influences ("Cultural differences between the examiner and the patient can greatly increase the risk of the examiner misinterpreting the patient's responses. For example, Waddell's signs are not valid in non-Anglo cultures, as their reliability has been tested only among English and North American patients.")[13(p27)]

Apply the Correct Causation Standard

The workers' compensation system arose in the early twentieth century, in response to tragedies like the Triangle Shirtwaist Factory fire.[2(p7),14] A grand bargain was struck between business and labor: workers and their families gave up the right to sue the employer for an injury or death, even when caused by employers' gross negligence. This protects employers from lawsuits and judgments that could bankrupt them. In exchange, the no-fault workers' compensation system was created to generally protect workers, guaranteeing them prompt medical care, partial wage replacement during their recovery, and limited compensation for permanent disabilities, for any injury "arising out of and in the course of employment."[2(pp7−8),15−17] As a result of this quid pro quo, the no-fault workers' compensation system uses a significantly different causation standard than physicians use in medical and scientific literature.

Physicians should be aware of how their jurisdiction has defined both the required degree of certainty, and the contribution threshold, when providing opinions related to causation. Attorneys and judges discredit or disregard medicolegal opinions that are not based on the legally defined standards.

In a medicolegal context, physicians should understand and analyze causation using the legally correct degree of certainty. The 95% probability standard used in evidence-based medicine is different from the 50.1% probability standard established in the law. Medical and scientific literature analyze cause based on P value,[18] requiring "the likelihood that an association between a potential cause and an effect to be greater than 95% for the relationship to be 'probable.' Everything else is only possible."[13(p25)] In contrast, the law defines the associations between an injury, incident, exposure, or employment and a condition to be "probable" if it is "more likely than not." Different jurisdictions or laws express the "more likely than not" concept through terms such as "reasonable degree of medical certainty," "reasonable degree of medical probability," or "more probable than not." Regardless of the terms used, the concept of medical probability in a legal context generally means a likelihood in excess of 50%, not the medical or scientific probability standard of 95%.[13(p25)] In some jurisdictions, an opinion based on medical "possibility" (less than 50% likelihood of a cause and effect relationship, but the causal relationship cannot be ruled out) is sufficient to establish causation, when combined with other nonmedical evidence supporting causation.

The law also establishes the extent or degree to which the injury, incident, exposure, or employment activity has contributed to a medical condition. The degree of contribution standard, can vary greatly among different jurisdictions and venues and often is dependent on case law defining what it means for an injury or condition to "arise out of" employment.[17] Different jurisdictions may require injured workers to prove that their employment or work injury is "the prevailing factor,"[19] "the major contributing cause,"[20] "a substantial contributing factor,"[21] "a causative factor,"[22] or a "more than negligible or theoretic"[23] factor in bringing about a condition. In some states, legal causation is established when preexisting conditions are "more than slightly" aggravated, exacerbated, accelerated, "lit up," or made symptomatic by employment or a work injury.[24] What constitutes "substantial," and the related role of preexisting conditions, varies widely.

Disability Is a Legal Determination, Decided by a Judge

Impairment is "a loss, loss of use, or derangement of any body part, organ system, or organ function."[25,26] Impairment ratings are meant to qualify and quantify the permanent functional impact of a medical condition on the individual to whom the rating is assigned. Therefore, the goal should be a rating system that accurately and reliably reflects impairment of a given individual and has a high level of inter-rater reliability.

As stated in the American Medical Association *Guides to the Evaluation of Permanent Impairment*, sixth edition, "Diagnosis should be evidence based, however, the impact of injury or illness is dependent on factors beyond physical and psychological aspects, including psychosocial, behavioral and contextual issues."[13(p9)] As discussed previously, not all persons with the same diagnosed condition end up with the exact same permanent outcome. Not all human beings are the same in terms of their capacities to endure, heal, and overcome. Not all people are provided the same level of care and treatment, nor do they all receive it timely or under the same optimal circumstances enabling the maximal recovery.

Disability is based on what a person can or cannot do after having an identified impairment. Disability, or what it means to be disabled, is a legal issue. Disability is defined differently in various legal contexts, depending on the idiosyncrasies of the applicable disability law or policy at issue (eg, 50 states' workers' compensation laws, the federal workers' compensation system,[27] Social Security disability insurance,[28] the Americans with Disabilities Act (ADA),[29] and the contractual terms of a disability policy). Generally, disability laws and policies set standards for measuring the effect of bodily impairment (physical or mental) on an individual's ability to perform tasks or jobs, which enables a person to be employable and self-supporting.

Disability is a legal determination rather than a medical determination. Nonmedical factors as well as variable legal definitions are considered in determining disability. Therefore, disability from a given diagnosis can be extremely different from person to person. A physician's assessment of impairment "must be further integrated with contextual information typically provided by nonphysician sources regarding psychological, social, vocational, and avocational issues" when determining disability.[13(p6)]

"Most physicians are not trained in assessing the full array of human functional activities and participations that are required for comprehensive disability determinations."[13(p5)] Limitations on an individual's function with respect to both activities of daily living and work activities are not objectively measurable. In determining disability, nonmedical factors, such as a person's age, education, work experience, transferrable skills, intellect, support network, and psychological resilience; the economy; and geographic area of residence, are all considerations. "The relationship between impairment and disability remains both complex and difficult, if not impossible, to predict."[13(p5)]

Physicians assign impairment ratings and perform disability assessments only in a medicolegal context. Ultimately, these expert opinions are meant to help a fact finder (jury, administrative law judge, or judge) understand the medical evidence and determine medical facts in issue.[30] Legally, the fact finder must analyze the medical facts, in combination with other legally relevant nonmedical facts, to determine whether or not and to what extent the legal definition of disability has been proved.

Accordingly, impairment ratings and medical disability assessments are tools used in a legal system. The tools are most helpful when they thoroughly describe and quantify the physiologic capabilities lost, and burdens added, as a result of an injury. This includes describing functional deficits, medically appropriate restrictions, and limitations on a person's residual physiologic capacity to perform tasks associated with work (eg, sit, stand, walk, kneel, crawl, bend, lift, twist, carry, squat, climb, push, pull, grasp, reach, make quotas, concentrate, understand, remember, adapt, decide, and interact).

This tool is even more helpful when it not only includes objectively manifested losses but also describes, and to the extent possible quantifies, subjective factors that could affect a person's ability to be gainfully employed (eg, losses of endurance, loss of pain-free function, need to alternate positions, need to take breaks, medication-related or pain-related interference with cognitive abilities and stamina, sleep interference due to pain, loss of coordination, burden of using prosthetics or medical appliances, need to miss work due to painful flare-ups or to seek treatment, and need to rely on family members for assistance). These factors are challenging to assess and can significantly burden injured workers or their families.[13(pp31–46)]

An evaluation that thoroughly describes and quantifies the physiologic capabilities lost, and burdens added, helps a fact finder analyze the impact of the physiologic impairment on the person's life, and assess whether any disability benefits are owed and, if so, how much. It helps injured workers realistically understand what they may or may not do, so that they can move forward with their life both at work and at home (eg, can no longer water ski but can go fishing). The information may help injured workers obtain reasonable accommodations under the ADA from their current employers, or from future employers, enabling them to keep working. It helps injured workers qualify for vocational retaining services, which enable them to retrain for a new line of work that is consistent with their residual capabilities. Ultimately, it helps the workers' compensation system, the civil justice system, the ADA, and the Social Security Administration, better accomplish their intended goals—and injured workers to move on with their lives.

SUMMARY

Injured workers deal with additional struggles while healing, forced on them by perceived and real problems within the workers' compensation system. The physician's role is critical in mitigating external complicating factors that can have a negative impact on recovery or prolong the process. The evaluating physician must recognize that legal causation differs from medical/scientific causation when opining on causation. Although physicians see individuals for disability evaluations or assessment, the determination of disability is a legal issue determined by a court. Disability evaluations are most useful when they thoroughly describe and quantify objectively manifested physiologic capabilities lost, added burdens, and subjective factors that could affect employability.

REFERENCES

1. Kelley JM, Kraft-Todd G, Schapira L, et al. The influence of the patient-clinician relationship on healthcare outcomes: a systematic review and meta-analysis of randomized controlled trials. PLoS One 2014;9(4):e94207. Available at: https://doi.org/10.1371/journal.pone.0094207. Accessed August 13, 2018.

2. U.S. Department of Labor. Does the workers' compensation system fulfill its obligations to injured workers? Washington, DC: U.S. Department of Labor; 2016. p. 13–23. Available at: https://www.dol.gov/asp/WorkersCompensationSystem/WorkersCompensationSystemReport.pdf. Accessed August 14, 2018.

3. Fagan KM, Hodgson MJ. Under-recording of work-related injuries and illnesses: an OSHA priority. J Safety Res 2016;60:79–83. Available at: https://doi.org/10. 1016/j.jsr.2016.12.002. Accessed August 10, 2018.

4. Grabel M. ProPublica. Berkes, H. NPR. The Demolition of Work Comp. In: Insult to injury, ProPublica March 4, 2015. NPR. 2015. Available at: https://www.propublica. org/article/the-demolition-of-workers-compensation. Accessed August 10, 2018.

5. Grabel M. The fallout of workers' comp 'reforms': 5 tales of harm. In: Insult to injury, ProPublica. 2015. Available at: https://www.propublica.org/article/ workers-compensation-injured-workers-share-stories-of-harm. Accessed August 10, 2018.

6. Grabel M. OSHA report echoes propublica and NPR's workers' comp findings. In: Insult to injury, ProPublica. 2015. Available at: https://www.propublica.org/article/ osha-report-echoes-propublica-and-nprs-workers-comp-findings. Accessed August 10, 2018.

7. OSHA. Adding inequality to injury: the costs of failing to protect workers on the job. Washington DC: U.S. Department of Labor; 2015. p. 2. Available at: https://www.osha.gov/Publications/inequality_michaels_june2015.pdf. Accessed August 10, 2018.

8. Spieler EA, Wagner GR. Counting matters: implications of undercounting in the BLS survey of occupational injuries and illnesses. Am J Ind Med 2014;57:1079.

9. Grabel M. All of this because somebody got hurt at work. In: Insult to injury, Pro-Publica. 2015. Available at: https://www.propublica.org/article/workers-comp-conferences-expos-and-middlemen. Accessed August 10, 2018.

10. Groopman J. How doctors think. New York: Houghton Mifflin Harcourt; 2007. p. 17.

11. American Psychiatric Association. Diagnostic and statistical manual of mental disorders. 5th edition. Arlington (VA): American Psychiatric Association; 2013. p. 321.

12. Main CJ, Waddell G. A reappraisal of the interpretation of "nonorganic signs.". Spine 1998;23(21):2367–71.

13. American Medical Association. Guides to the evaluation of permanent impairment. 6th edition. Chicago: American Medical Association; 2008.

14. The Triangle Shirtwaist Factory Fire. OSHA, U.S. Department of Labor. Available at: https://www.osha.gov/oas/trianglefactoryfire.html. Accessed August 12, 2018.

15. Baker v. Bridgestone/Firestone & Old Republic Ins., 872 N.W.2d 672, 676-679 (Iowa 2015).

16. Mclarin CF, Baldwin M. Workers' compensation: benefits, coverage, and costs 2015. Washington, DC: National Academy of Social Insurance; 2017.

17. Larson A, Larson L. Ch. 3-10. Larson's workers' compensation desk edition, vol. 1. Danver (MA): Matthew Bender & Co. Inc; 2002.

18. American Medical Association. Guides to the evaluation of disease and injury causation. 2nd edition. Chicago: American Medical Association; 2014. p. 26–7.

19. See e.g. Mo. Rev. Stat. §287.020 (2017).

20. See e.g. 56 O.R.S. §656.005(7)(a)(A) (2017).

21. See e.g. Gist v. Atlas Staffing, 910 N.W.2d 24, 29-31 (Minn. 2018).

22. See e.g. Sisbro, Inc. v. Industrial Commission, et. al, 797 N.E.2d 655, 207 Ill. 2d 193, 278 Ill. Dec 70 (Ill. 2003).

23. See e.g. S. Coast Framing, Inc. v. Workers' Comp. Appeals Bd., 61 Cal. 4th 291, 298, 188 Cal. Rptr. 3d 46, 51, 349 P.3d 141, 146 (2015).

24. See e.g. Ziegler v. U.S. Gypsum Co., 106 N.W.2d 591, 598 (Iowa 1960); Rose v. John Deere Ottumwa Works, 76 N.W.2d 756, 761 (Iowa 1956).

25. American Medical Association. Guides to the evaluation of permanent impairment. 5th edition. Chicago: American Medical Association; 2001. 2.

26. American Medical Association. Guides to the evaluation of permanent impairment. 4th edition. Chicago: American Medical Association; 1993.

27. Federal Employees' Compensation Act (FECA), ch. 458, 39 Stat. 742 (1916), 5 U.S.C. §§ 8101-8193 (2013) (codified as amended in scattered sections of 1 U.S.C., 5 U.S.C., and 18 U.S.C.). Available at: https://www.dol.gov/owcp/dfec/regs/statutes/feca.htm. Accessed August 14, 2018.

28. Title II, Federal Old-Age, Survivors, and Disability Insurance Benefits, 42 USC §§401-434. 20 C.F.R. §§404.1-404.2127. Available at: https://www.ssa.gov/OP_Home/ssact/title02/0200.htm; https://www.ssa.gov/OP_Home/cfr20/404/404-0000.htm. Accessed August 14, 2018.

29. Americans with Disabilities Act of 1990 (ADA), 42 U.S.C. §§ 12101-12213 (2013) (amended 2008).

30. See e.g. Federal Rule of Evidence 702.

Common Metrics for Impairment Ratings

Christopher R. Brigham, MD, MMS

KEYWORDS

- Impairment • Disability • AMA *Guides to the Evaluation of Permanent Impairment*
- Whole person

KEY POINTS

- Impairment reflects a "a significant deviation, loss, or loss of use of any body structure or body function in an individual with a health condition, disorder, or disease."
- Disability refers to "activity limitations and/or participation restrictions in an individual with a health condition, disorder, or disease."
- Impairment and disability are not synonymous; however, some workers' compensation jurisdictions use permanent impairment ratings to define permanent partial disability awards.
- The American Medical Association *Guides to the Evaluation of Permanent Impairment* (AMA *Guides*) have evolved from their origin in 1971, with the current standard the sixth edition. The sixth edition uses the framework based on the International Classification of Functioning, Disability and Health.
- Impairment rating values will change and currently are based largely on consensus. Future research could use empirical evidence on the relationship between impairment ratings and earnings losses to improve the ability of the AMA *Guides* to predict the economic consequences of a disabling injury.

INTRODUCTION

Impairment is defined in the American Medical Association *Guides to the Evaluation of Permanent Impairment*, sixth edition (AMA *Guides*), as "a significant deviation, loss, or loss of use of any body structure or body function in an individual with a health condition, disorder, or disease."[1] According to the AMA *Guides*, permanent impairments are assessed when a patient is at maximum medical improvement, the point at which a condition has stabilized and is unlikely to change (improve or worsen) substantially in the next year, with or without treatment. The AMA *Guides* are the most widely used

Disclosure Statement: Editor, American Medical Association *Guides Newsletter*, and Senior Contributing Editor, American Medical Association *Guides to the Evaluation of Permanent Impairment*.
Brigham and Associates, Inc., Hilton Head Island, SC, USA
E-mail address: cbrigham@cbrigham.com

Phys Med Rehabil Clin N Am 30 (2019) 533–540
https://doi.org/10.1016/j.pmr.2019.03.003
1047-9651/19/© 2019 Elsevier Inc. All rights reserved.

standard for defining impairment and used in the workers' compensation arena (state and federal) and also some automobile casualty and personal injury cases.

The World Health Organization (WHO) definition of impairment is "any loss or abnormality of psychological, physiologic or anatomic structure or function."[2] The Social Security Administration defines this as "an impairment that results from anatomical, physiological, or psychological abnormalities which can be shown by medically acceptable clinical and laboratory diagnostic techniques" and the impairment "must be established by medical evidence consisting of signs, symptoms, and laboratory findings—not only by the individual's statement of symptoms."[3]

With the AMA *Guides*, impairment is reflected in a numeric rating that may be to the whole person (ranging from 0% = no impairment to 100% = death) and/or to regional impairments (upper extremity, hand, digits, lower extremity, foot/ankle, and/or toes), which are scheduled to the body part and can be converted to a percentage of the whole person if allowed. It is essential that there is a valid and reliable metric for assessing impairment.

A defined standard is required to achieve valid and reliable impairment ratings.

IMPAIRMENT VERSUS DISABILITY

Impairment is not synonymous with disability, which is defined in the AMA *Guides* as "activity limitations and/or participation restrictions in an individual with a health condition, disorder, or disease." The WHO defines disability as an activity limitation that creates a difficulty in the performance, accomplishment, or completion of an activity in the manner or within the range considered normal for a human being.

Whether or not an impairment results in an occupational disability depends on many factors, including how the impairment may result in functional loss, functional demands for an activity, resiliency, and motivation, both for the individual and for others in accommodating that individual. An individual may have minimal impairment yet be disabled occupationally, for example, a concert pianist with a hand injury. Someone may have marked impairment and continue to work, for example, an attorney who is wheelchair bound.

An impairment rating is a necessary component of any disability determination but not the sole nor necessarily adequate determinant. The impairment rating system is that part of a disability evaluation that is most amenable to and dependent on a physician's assessment. The AMA *Guides* explain that impairment ratings are a physician-driven first approximation of a process that attempts to link impairment with a quantitative estimate of functional losses in the patient's "personal sphere of activity" or activities of daily living (ADLs). Inclusion of ADLs is important because they serve as the preferred functional metric for physicians who frequently communicate about severity of impairment (the medical condition) in terms of how it interferes with the ADLs of a particular affected patient. For example, an individual with disabling hip pain associated with end-stage (bone-on-bone) arthritis might have particular difficulties abducting and externally rotating the affected hip and expressed simply as the inability to cross the legs to tie a shoe on the affected side.

Metrics exist to a varying degree, to calculate losses to the impaired individual in terms of work disability (loss of earnings and/or earning capacity) but also for nonwork disability (losses in ability to pursue hobbies, recreation, and so forth) and quality of life (eg, losses in terms of medical burden of care, life satisfaction, and other areas).[4] A case-control study of 21,663 workers' compensation claimants in California with impairment ratings based on the AMA *Guides*, fifth edition, demonstrated that impairment ratings are accurate predictors of disability severity on average, but their ability to measure disability could be improved with additional information on how the relationship between ratings and earnings loss varies according to patient and injury characteristics.[5] Otherwise, there are few studies and fewer methodologically sound studies that have compared impairment ratings to disability and/or appropriate compensation.

Despite impairment and disability being different, some systems use a permanent impairment rating as a direct proxy for permanent partial disability.[6] Impairment ratings are not intended, however, to measure disability nor are they intended to directly predict economic compensation for disability. Other systems may use a formula where impairment and other factors, such as age and occupation, are used to define permanent partial disability. Jurisdictions need to have sufficient knowledge about the relationship between impairment ratings, benefit levels, and earnings losses to make informed choices about the socially desirable benefit levels.

HISTORY OF THE AMERICAN MEDICAL ASSOCIATION *GUIDES TO THE EVALUATION OF PERMANENT IMPAIRMENT*

The AMA *Guides* are a standardized objective reference and reporting guide originally published in 1971 and periodically updated and revised to the current sixth edition, published in 2007. Revisions replaced outdated approaches and information with current data and consensus. The application of this updating approach, however, has not been universally adopted by virtual of interests of certain stakeholders, local preferences, legislative mandate, and/or other barriers.

The AMA *Guides* started in 1958 with publication of an article, "A Guide to the Evaluation of Permanent Impairment of the Extremities and Back."[7] In 1971, a compendium of 13 guides became the first edition.[8] The second edition[9] was published 13 years later in 1984, and the third edition[10] was published in 1988. The third edition was the first to use the Swanson[11] methodology, which assigned discrete impairment ratings to specific range-of-motion deficits of the upper extremities. It was replaced 2 years later by the third edition, revised.[12] The fourth edition,[13] published in 1993, provided many refinements, including a diagnosis-related estimate (DRE) or injury model for evaluation of spinal injuries, alternative approaches to assessing lower extremity impairment, and a pain chapter. The DRE model was unique in allowing for assignment of an impairment rating based solely on the diagnosis, even if maximum medical improvement had not yet been reached. The fifth edition,[14] published in 2000, was nearly twice the size of its predecessor. It provided more detailed directives in all chapters and modified the approaches used for spinal impairment evaluation by providing guidance on the choice of the rating method and the impairment ranges for DRE categories. The sixth edition represents a continued evolution in impairment evaluation.

Previous editions were criticized for several reasons, including use of confusing, inconsistent, and antiquated terminology of disablement; ratings that failed to reflect perceived or actual loss of function; validity and reliability of ratings that were questionable; and lack of internal consistency.[15,16] In response to these criticisms, the following changes were recommended:

- Standardize assessment of ADLs limitations associated with physical impairments.
- Apply functional assessment tools to validate impairment rating scales.
- Include measures of functional loss in the impairment rating.
- Improve overall intrarater and interrater reliability and internal consistency.

Studies comparing previous editions of the AMA *Guides* have demonstrated poor interrater reliability and revealed that many impairment ratings are incorrect and often rated significantly higher than is appropriate.[17]

The AMA *Guides* create the opportunity for consistency of impairment ratings among physicians. As a result, there is an opportunity for reduction in friction costs arising within the compensations systems, speedy resolution, and fairness to all stakeholders.[18]

AMERICAN MEDICAL ASSOCIATION *GUIDES TO THE EVALUATION OF PERMANENT IMPAIRMENT*, SIXTH EDITION

The sixth edition provide a consistent, well-defined methodology to enhance the relevancy of impairment ratings, improve internal consistency, promote greater precision, and standardize the rating process. A goal was to provide an impairment rating guide that is authoritative, fair, and equitable to all parties. The 5 new axioms of the sixth edition are presented in **Box 1**.

Clinical discussions among physician colleagues regarding potential severity of an illness or injury typically involve 4 basic points of consideration:

1. What is the problem (diagnosis)?
2. What symptoms and resulting functional difficulty does the patient report?
3. What are the physical findings pertaining to the problem?
4. What are the results of clinical studies?

These same basic considerations are used by physicians to evaluate and communicate about impairment. The sixth edition expands the spectrum of diagnoses recognized in impairment rating, considers functional consequences of the impairment as a part of each physician's detailed history, and clarifies significant physical examination findings and clinical testing.

The sixth edition uses the framework based on the International Classification of Functioning, Disability and Health (ICF), a comprehensive model of disablement developed by the WHO. This framework is intended for describing and measuring health and disability at the individual and population levels and is illustrated in **Fig. 1**. The ICF is a classification of health and health-related domains that describe body functions and structures, activities, and participation. The domains are classified from body, individual, and societal perspectives. The ICF

Box 1
Five axioms of the American Medical Association *Guides to the Evaluation of Permanent Impairment*, sixth edition

1. The AMA *Guides* adopt the terminology and conceptual framework of disablement as put forward by ICF.

2. The AMA *Guides* become more diagnosis based with these diagnoses evidence based when possible.

3. Simplicity, ease-of-application, and following precedent, where applicable, are given high priority, with the goal of optimizing interrater and intrarater reliability.

4. Rating percentages derived according to the AMA *Guides* are functionally based, to the fullest practical extent possible.

5. The AMA *Guides* stress conceptual and methodological congruity within and between organ system ratings.

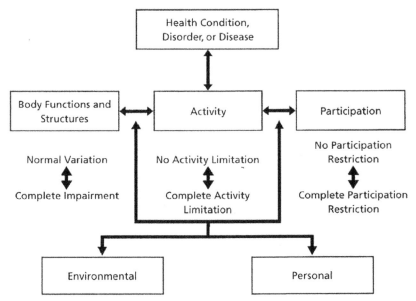

Fig. 1. ICF model of disablement.

systematically groups different domains for a person with a given health condition (eg, what a person with a disease or disorder does do or can do). *Functioning* is an umbrella term encompassing all body functions, activities, and participations; similarly, *disability* serves as an umbrella term for impairments, activity limitations, or participation restrictions. Because an individual's functioning and disability occurs in a context, the ICF also includes a list of contextual (eg, environmental and/or personal) factors. The ICF model reflects the dynamic interactions between an individual with a given health condition, and the environment and personal factors that have an impact on the resulting activity limitations and participation restrictions in any given case.

Using the analytic framework of the ICF, the sixth edition defined 5 impairment classes that permit the rating of the patient from no impairment to most severe. Diagnosis-based grids were developed for each organ system, which use commonly accepted consensus-based criteria to classify most diagnoses relevant to a particular organ or body part into 5 classes of impairment severity ranging from class 0 (normal) to class 5 (very severe). The final impairment is determined by adjusting the initial impairment rating by factors that may include physical findings, the results of clinical tests, and functional reports by the patient. The basic template of the diagnosis-based grid is common to each organ system and chapter. Although there is variation in the ancillary factors used to develop the impairment rating (depending on the body part), there is greater internal consistency between chapters than was formerly seen.

The sixth edition is composed of 17 chapters. Chapter 1, "Conceptual Foundations and Philosophy," and Chapter 2, "Practical Applications of the Guides," define the overall approaches to assessing impairment. Most impairment ratings are performed for musculoskeletal painful conditions; therefore, the most commonly used chapters are Chapter 15, "The Upper Extremities, Chapter 16, "The Lower Extremities," and Chapter 17, "The Spine and Pelvis."

IMPAIRMENT RATING VALUES

Impairment ratings should reflect real outcomes and be based, to the greatest extent possible, on scientific evidence or, when this is lacking, expert consensus. Most impairment rating values at this time are based on legal precedent and expert consensus derived by using a modified Delphi process. With changes in approaches among different editions of the AMA *Guides*, changes in impairment rating values will occur.

A comparative analysis of AMA *Guides* ratings by the fourth, fifth, and sixth editions was performed by assessing 200 cases.[19] The clinical data were used to determine the resulting whole person permanent impairment (WPI) according to each of these 3 editions. The average WPI per case was 4.82% WPI per the sixth edition, 6.33% WPI per the fifth edition, and 5.5% WPI per the fourth edition. The overall average WPI for each diagnosis was 3.53% WPI per the sixth edition, 4.59% WPI per the fifth edition, and 4.00% WPI per the fourth edition. This analysis revealed a statistically significant difference between average whole person impairment ratings when comparing the sixth edition with the fifth edition but not when comparing the sixth edition results with those of the fourth edition.

With advancements in medical and surgical technology, expected functional outcomes have improved enabling decreasing impairment ratings in many situations. For example, the default impairment for a total knee replacement with a good result was previously rated as 50% lower extremity impairment with the fourth edition (published in 1993) and subsequent fifth edition (published in 2000); however, in the sixth edition, this was reduced to 37% lower extremity impairment to reflect the advances in medical science and associated improved outcomes for this particular condition.

Revisions in specific impairment values assigned for certain conditions occurred in preparing the sixth edition. For example, in the fifth edition, a single-level cervical fusion would result in a 25% to 28% WPI; yet, these patients typically have excellent functional results; however, this impairment was consistent with that given for a below-knee amputation. In contrast, patients with intractable cervical radiculopathy, much more impairing and disabling, were limited to 15% to 18% WPI according to the fifth edition. Modifications in approaches to determining impairment ratings also are required. The goal of any medical or surgical intervention should be to improve the level of functioning and well-being of the patient. Yet, using the fifth edition, patients often receive greater impairment for spinal surgical interventions. In the fourth edition, ratings for "surgery to treat an impairment does not modify the original impairment estimate, which remains the same in spite of any changes in signs or symptoms that may follow the surgery." (fourth ed, p100) Thus a patient with a cervical radiculopathy who had a cervical fusion would have received a 15% WPI using the fourth edition (because surgery was not considered and the patient was rated on the presenting problem, not the outcome), a 25% to 28% WPI using the fifth edition (because surgery was considered), and a 6% WPI with the sixth edition (because impairment is based primarily on the outcome.)

Over time, certain approaches are found not valid and/or not reliable. For example, range of motion no longer is used to assess spinal impairment, because current evidence does not support this as a reliable indicator of specific pathology or permanent functional loss.

Changes in impairment values should be expected and welcomed. If ratings change and are part of a formula used to reach a benefit payment, benefits will change as well. The solution is for jurisdiction and legislators to frequently assess their benefit structure so that all factors, including impairment ratings, are taken into consideration when determining levels of compensation. The common goal that all stakeholders share is for an injured person to receive appropriate and effective care that results in the fullest possible restoration of function in a particular case. The ideal outcome short of no impairment and no disability is the one that enables maximal functional recovery and enables a fair determination of residual disability that cannot be totally eliminated in most cases.

FUTURE

Approaches to impairment and disability assessment will continue to evolve. It is imperative that all stakeholders understand the differences between ratings of impairment and disability. Future research could use empirical evidence on the relationship between impairment ratings and earnings losses to hopefully improve the ability of the AMA *Guides* to predict the economic consequences of an illness or injury as part of the larger disability determination process in which the health care provider is partially engaged.

REFERENCES

1. American Medical Association. Guides to the evaluation of permanent impairment. 3rd edition. Chicago: American Medical Association; 2008. p. 611.
2. World Health Organization. International classification of functioning, disability and health: ICF. Geneva (Switzerland): World Health Organization; 2001. Available at: http://www.who.int/classifications/icf/en/.
3. Social Security Administration. Program Operations Manual System, Part 04, Disability Insurance. Office of the Federal Register. Available at: https://secure.ssa.gov/apps10/. Accessed May 14, 2019.
4. Rondinelli RD, Eskay-Auerbach M, Ranavaya MI, et al. AMA guides to the evaluation of permanent impairment, sixth edition: a response to the NCCI study. AMA Guides Newsletter 2012.
5. Seabury SA, Neuhauser F, Nuckols T. American Medical Association impairment ratings and earnings losses due to disability. J Occup Environ Med 2013;55(3):286–91.
6. Burton JF. Workers' compensation cash benefits: part one: the building blocks. In: Workers compensation policy review. 2008. p. 15–28.
7. American Medical Association. A guide to the evaluation of permanent impairment of the extremities and back. JAMA 1958;166(suppl):1–122.
8. American Medical Association. Guides to the evaluation of permanent impairment. 1st edition. Chicago: American Medical Association; 1971.
9. American Medical Association. Guides to the evaluation of permanent impairment. 2nd edition. Chicago: American Medical Association; 1984.
10. American Medical Association. Guides to the evaluation of permanent impairment. 3rd edition. Chicago: American Medical Association; 1988.
11. Swanson AB. Evaluation of impairment of function in the hand. Surg Clin North Am 1964;44:925–40.
12. American Medical Association. Guides to the evaluation of permanent impairment. 3rd edition revised. Chicago: American Medical Association; 1990.
13. American Medical Association. Guides to the evaluation of permanent impairment. 4th edition. Chicago: American Medical Association; 1993.
14. American Medical Association. Guides to the evaluation of permanent impairment. 5th edition. Chicago: American Medical Association; 2000.

15. Spieler EA, Barth PS, Burton JF, et al. Recommendations to guide revision of the guides to the evaluation of permanent impairment. JAMA 2000;283(4):519–23.
16. Rondinelli RD, Katz RT. Merits and shortcomings of the American Medical Association Guides to the evaluation of permanent impairment, 5th edition: a physiatric perspective. Phys Med Rehabil Clin N Am 2002;13:355–70.
17. Burton JF. Workers' compensation cash benefits: part one: the building blocks. In: Workers Compensation Policy Review. Workers' Disability Income Systems, Inc. March/April 2008. p. 15–28.
18. Brigham CR, Uehlein WF, Uejo C, et al. Impairment rating insights. AMA Guides Newsletter 2008.
19. Brigham CR, Uejo C, McEntire A, et al. Comparative analysis of AMA guides ratings by the fourth, fifth and sixth editions. AMA Guides Newsletter 2010.

Evaluating Return-to-work Ability Using Functional Capacity Evaluation

E. Randolph Soo Hoo, MD, MPH

KEYWORDS

- RTW assessment • Employers • Fitness of Duty

KEY POINTS

- It is beneficial for both the worker and employer for the worker to return to work early as possible after an illness, injury, or prolonged absence.
- Because employers are ultimately responsible for the return to work decision, a medical RTW assessment is commonly required to assure that the worker is medically able to and physically capable of performing the job tasks.
- Consequently, many employers depend on the opinions from medical providers.
- Valid FCEs can provide objective measurements of work-related strength capabilities and are useful in supporting a medical provider's opinion of a worker's ability to RTW or FFD.

The longer a worker is absent from work due an injury or illness, the more difficult it is for the worker to return to work.[1–3] The longer a worker is away from work, the greater financial burden placed on the employer due to productivity loss, insurance costs, and other business-related costs.[4–6] Therefore, it is within the best interest for both the worker and the employer that a worker returns to work as early as possible after an illness, injury, or prolonged absence.[7–9]

Administratively, the final decision to allow the worker to return to work is borne by the employer. Consequently, many employers pursue assurances by means of a medical return to work (RTW), fitness for duty (FFD), and related work assessments to verify the worker has no medical contraindications for returning to work and that the worker is physically capable of performing the physical demands of the job. Although the medical provider's authority is not matched with the final authority for returning to work, the provider is relied on for their input.

Conceptually, the medical RTW process is similar to 1-dimensional linear disability models[10,11] in which the impact of a medical condition is assessed, a determination made for the presence of any consequential medical restrictions or functional

The author has nothing to disclose.
Medical Dimensions, One South Church, Suite 1200, Tucson, AZ 85701, USA
E-mail address: rsoohoo191@aol.com

Phys Med Rehabil Clin N Am 30 (2019) 541–559
https://doi.org/10.1016/j.pmr.2019.04.002
pmr.theclinics.com

limitations, recommendations offered for accommodations necessary to mitigate restrictions or limitations, and an administrative decision for disability or RTW is made (**Fig. 1**).

As with employers bearing the responsibility for the final return to work determination, the medical provider is accountable for the medical determination of the worker's medical and physical fitness to return to work.[12,13] Determining the worker's medical fitness to return to work necessitates an understanding of the underlying medical impairment and how it affects the worker's ability to return to work.[14,15] Unfortunately, depending on the medical provider's expertise, comfort level on offering an opinion, and/or personal biases, there is variability in the opinions among different providers.[16–19] Although many medical providers formulate their medical opinions based on intuitive conjectures, there are resources (ie, functional capacity evaluations [FCEs]) available to the provider to help formulate an objective opinion of the worker's medical fitness to return to work.

Although there are many psychological and other physiologic considerations, this article focuses on strength considerations related to physical activities for industrial material handling (ie, the movement and handling of materials).

WHAT IS FUNCTION? TERMS AND CONCEPTS

Medicolegal experts and medical providers are responsible for translating and communicating functional ability, related to a worker's health condition, easily understood by the employer and others.[20–22] To do so, the medical provider must understand commonly used terms and concepts employers and others are familiar with.

In the United States, there are 2 commonly used taxonomy systems incorporating function descriptors within their respective classification schemes: the US Department of Labor's Dictionary of Occupational Titles (DOT) and the Occupational Information Network (O*NET). Whereas O*NET is in widespread use in the vocational analysis

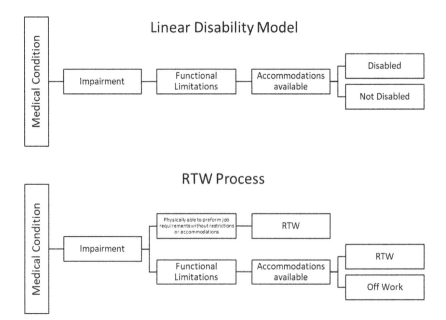

Fig. 1. RTW process similarities to linear disability model.

setting, DOT remains in widespread use in settings for Workers' Compensation, US Equal Employment Opportunity Commission, and other arenas.

Dictionary of Occupational Titles

The US Department of Labor published the DOT in 1938 to assist employers, government officials, and vocational analysts to evaluate and catalog different occupations. Focus is placed on occupational requirements, not what is required of the worker. To do so, DOT used occupation-specific information based on 23 physical functional elements and 5 mental functional elements of work to describe occupations in the national economy.[23,24] Using the physical functional elements, DOT classified occupations by physical work demand levels.

Physical requirements of the occupation are assessed in terms of exertion, posture, manipulation, and sensory functions (**Table 1**).

Manual material handing exertion thresholds for lifting, carrying, pulling, or pushing are used to define physical work levels: "Negligible," 10 pounds, 20 pounds, 50 pounds, and 100 pounds. The frequency (ie, occasional, frequent, and constant) the exertions are then used to categorize occupation physical work demand levels: Sedentary Work, Light Work, Medium Work, Heavy Work, and Very Heavy Work levels[23,25,26] (**Fig. 2**):

Sedentary Work: exerting up to 10 pounds of force occasionally

Light Work: exerting up to 20 pounds of force occasionally, and/or up to 10 pounds of force frequently, and/or a negligible amount of force constantly

Medium Work: exerting 20 to 50 pounds of force occasionally, and/or 10 to 25 pounds of force frequently, and/or greater than negligible up to 10 pounds of force constantly to move objects.

Heavy Work: exerting 50 to 100 pounds of force occasionally, and/or 25 to 50 pounds of force frequently, and/or 10 to 20 pounds of force constantly to move objects.

Very Heavy Work: exerting in excess of 100 pounds of force occasionally, and/or in excess of 50 pounds of force frequently, and/or in excess of 20 pounds of force constantly to move objects.

Occasionally is defined as an activity or condition that exists up to one-third of the time. Frequently is an activity or condition occurring from one-third to two-thirds of the time. "Of the time" is ambiguous and has been generally regarded as applicable to an 8-hour work day. However, others have considered this as referencing portions of a work shift (eg, number of times per hour). Moreover, the frequency descriptors are not used for sitting, standing, or walking tolerances (**Table 2**).

Vocationally, the physical work demands levels are refined using nonmaterial handling factors (see **Table 2**). Except for Very Heavy Work, the physical demands work levels are adjusted using nonmaterial handling physical elements.[27,28] If, for example, a worker is considered in the medium work level (lifting/carrying 50 pounds occasionally, 20 pounds frequently, or 10 pounds constantly), but cannot frequently stoop or crouch, the worker is vocationally considered in the Light Work category.

Occupational Information Network

DOT was deemed obsolete by the U.S. Department of Labor and was replaced by O*NET in the 1990s.[29–32] Occupations from 1938 to the 1990s were reclassified and newer occupations since 1997 are classified using O*NET terminology.[33] Although obsolete, DOT terminology remains embedded in the traditional framework describing

Table 1
DOT physical functional elements of work

Strength		Postural		Manipulative		Sensory	
Lifting	Raising or lowering an object form one height to another	Climbing	Traveling vertical distance using feet, legs, hands, or arms	Reaching	Extension of hands and arms in all directions including overhead	Talking	Communication of concepts through spoken words
Carrying	Horizontal transport of an object using hands, arms, or shoulders	Balancing	Maintaining body balance to prevent falls while walking, standing, crouching, and so forth	Handling	Grasping, holding, or manipulation of an object using the hand or hands	Hearing	Perception of sound through the ears
Pushing	Movement of an object away from the force	Stooping	Forward bending at the waist	Fingering	Pinching, picking, or manipulation an object with fingers	Tasting	Distinguishing flavors or tastes
Pulling	Movement of an object in the direction of the force	Kneeling	Maintaining a vertical position with weight bearing on one or both knees	Feeling	Perception of an object's size, shape, temperature, texture, and so forth	Smelling	Distinguishing of odors or smells using nose
Standing	Maintaining vertical position on feet without moving about	Crouching	Forward and downward bending with flexion at both waist and knees			Vision	Perception of light to distinguish objects through near acuity, far acuity, depth perception, accommodation, color vision, and field of vision
Walking	Horizontal motion using feet	Crawling	Horizontal motion with propulsion using hands and knees or feet				
Sitting	Maintain seated position						
Controls	Use of upper or lower extremities for hand-arm or foot-leg controls						

Data from Selected characteristics of occupations defined in the revised dictionary of occupational titles, Revised 4th Edition Appendix C Physical Demands, 1993; U.S. Government Printing Office Superintendent of Documents, Mail Stop: SSOP, Washington, DC 20402-9328;C1-C4 and 20 CFR § 404.1567 Physical exertion requirements.

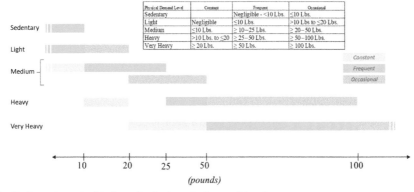

Fig. 2. Department of Labor physical work demand levels.

Table 2				
Nonexertional determinants affecting DOT work levels				
Work Activity	**Sedentary**	**Light Work**	**Medium Work**	**Heavy Work**
Sitting	Maximum 2 h continuously; total of 6 of 8 h	6 of 8 h totally; minimum of 2 h continuously	6 of 8 h totally; minimum of 2 h continuously	6 of 8 h totally; minimum of 2 h continuously
Stand/walk	Short distances without aids	6 of 8 h without aids	6 of 8 h without aids	6 of 8 h without aids
Hand use	Fine manipulation/ gross hand line	N/A	N/A	N/A
Stoop/crouch	Occasionally[a]	Occasionally[a]	Frequently[b]	Frequently[b]
Climb/kneel crouch/ balance	N/A	Specific job requirements	Specific job requirements (at least occasionally)	Specific job requirements
Push/pull	N/A	20 lb without bending/50 lb on wheels	30 lb without bending/75 lb on wheels	50 lb without bending/100 lb on wheels
Upper extremities	N/A	Reach overhead; manipulate fingers; handle gross objects	Reach overhead; manipulate fingers; handle gross objects	N/A
Lower extremities	N/A	Repetitive foot use	Repetitive foot use	N/A
Environment	N/A	N/A	No severe limitations	No severe limitations

[a] Occasionally = Activity up to 33% of the time.
[b] Frequently = Activity from 33% to 66% of the time.
Data from Selected characteristics of occupations defined in the revised dictionary of occupational titles, Revised 4th Edition Appendix C Physical Demands, 1993; U.S. Government Printing Office Superintendent of Documents, Mail Stop: SSOP, Washington, DC 20402-9328;C1-C4 and 20 CFR § 404.1567 Physical exertion requirements.

occupations for RTW or FFD purposes, it is incumbent on the medical expert to understand O*NET terms and principles.

O*NET is a digital only online relational database created to provide occupational information in response to the constant changes reflecting occupational requirements, worker attributes, and societal employment needs. Unlike the DOT, O*NET does not categorize occupations by physical or mental functional levels. Instead, O*NET uses 275 descriptors to classify job families (jobs with similar characteristics or traits) based on what is required of the job and what is required of the worker (**Fig. 3**).[34,35]

For each occupation, O*NET provides information regarding:

- Worker experience: training, experience, and applicable certifications needed for the work
- Worker requirements and characteristics: skills and knowledge required of the occupation
- Worker characteristics: abilities, interests, and personal values needed to perform the work
- Occupation requirements: generalized work activity and context within the organizational structure
- Occupation-specific requirements: knowledge and skills
- Labor market information: occupational outlook and pay scale

The O*NET database does not incorporate the Sedentary, Light, Medium, Heavy, or Very Heavy physical work demand levels used in the DOT. O*NET does not use frequency descriptors such as occasional or frequent. Rather than listing physical factors as strength, postural, manipulation, and sensory functions, O*NET focuses the physical aspects of the job in terms of psychomotor abilities, endurance, flexibility, balance, coordination, and sensory abilities[36] (**Table 3**).

Unlike DOT, O*NET considers not only occupation requirements, but also what is required of the worker. Elements relating to physical abilities are expressed as

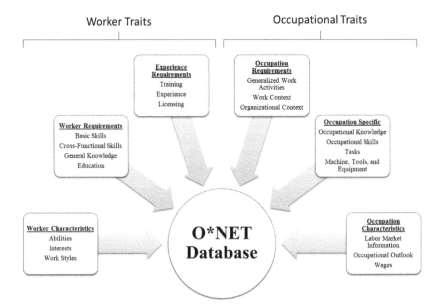

Fig. 3. O*NET content model.

Table 3
O*NET physical factors

Psychomotor Abilities — Abilities that Influence the Capacity to Manipulate and Control Objects	Endurance — The Ability to Exert Oneself Physically over Long Periods Without Getting out of Breath	Flexibility, Balance, and Coordination — Abilities Related to the Control of Gross Body Movements	Sensory Abilities — Abilities that Influence Visual, Auditory, and Speech Perception
Fine manipulative abilities — Abilities related to the manipulation of objects	Stamina — The ability to exert yourself physically over long periods of time without getting winded or out of breath	Extent flexibility — The ability to bend, stretch, twist, or reach with your body, arms, and/or legs	Visual abilities — Abilities related to visual sensory input
Control movement abilities — Abilities related to the control and manipulation of objects in time and space		Dynamic flexibility — The ability to quickly and repeatedly bend, stretch, twist, or reach out with your body, arms, and/or legs	Auditory and speech abilities — Abilities related to auditory and oral input
Reaction time and speed abilities — Abilities related to speed of manipulation of objects		Gross body coordination — The ability to coordinate the movement of your arms, legs, and torso together when the whole body is in motion	
Physical abilities — Abilities that influence strength, endurance, flexibility, balance, and coordination		Gross body equilibrium — The ability to keep or regain your body balance or stay upright when in an unstable position	
Trunk strength — The ability to use your abdominal and lower back muscles to support part of the body repeatedly or continuously overt me without "giving out" or fatiguing			

dynamic flexibility, dynamic strength, explosive strength, extent flexibility, gross body coordination, gross body equilibrium, stamina, static strength, and trunk strength (**Table 4**).[37] Physical abilities are described in the context of the importance of what is needed for the activity on Likert-type scales for the importance, level, and extent of the activity.[38]

FUNCTIONAL CAPACITY EVALUATIONS

Matching a worker's physical capacity to their ability to complete real-world manual material handling tasks is premised on determining or measuring the worker's functional capacity and comparing the demonstrated capacity to the physical requirements of the job.[39] Rather than relying on speculation, a properly designed and conducted FCE can provide the medical provider more objective insight into a worker's physical ability to return to work.[40,41]

FCEs are systematic approaches used to evaluate a worker's ability to carry out meaningful tasks.[42] FCE uses known metrics about the physical demands of a work task (ie, forces required for material handling, material displacements, body positions) and translates the worker's demonstrated capacity into constructs to which the worker or incumbent population can be matched. In other words, FCEs are useful for matching a worker's demonstrated capacity to what is required of the work task. If the worker demonstrates the ability to complete an FCE task relative to the actual work task, an inference can be made that the individual can safely perform that work task.

Using FCEs to augment a medical RTW or an FFD opinion can be confusing to the medical provider because there is no standardized strategy to globally assess function and because there is no consistency among the vast number of different FCE systems on how the interpret measurements.[43–45] This poses an issue, especially in the

Table 4
O*NET physical abilities characteristic

Physical Ability	Description
Dynamic flexibility	Ability to quickly and repeatedly bend, stretch, twist, or reach out with your body, arms, and/or legs
Dynamic strength	Ability to exert muscle force repeatedly or continuously over time. This involves muscular endurance and resistance to muscle fatigue
Explosive strength	Ability to use short bursts of muscle force to propel oneself (as in jumping or sprinting), or to throw an object
Extent flexibility	Ability to bend, stretch, twist, or reach with your body, arms, and/or legs
Gross body coordination	Ability to coordinate the movement of your arms, legs, and torso together when the whole body is in motion
Gross body equilibrium	Ability to keep or regain your body balance or stay upright when in an unstable position
Stamina	Ability to exert yourself physically over long periods of time without getting winded or out of breath
Static strength	Ability to exert maximum muscle force to lift, push, pull, or carry objects
Trunk strength	Ability to use your abdominal and lower back muscles to support part of the body repeatedly or continuously over time without "giving out" or fatiguing

medicolegal setting, because results from 2 independent FCE providers on the same subject can result in substantially different findings.

Most FCEs attempt to align findings to DOT physical work demands levels (see **Fig. 2**), but seldom consider the nonexertional work components (see **Table 2**). FCEs rarely address the more contemporary physical characteristics found in O*NET (see **Table 3**). Although professional organizations such as the American Physical Therapy Association and the American Occupational Therapy Association offer guidance on the use of FCEs findings and suggest what should be considered to match a worker to a job, there is no uniform guidance addressing which work tasks are measured or how they are obtained, nor are there standardized guidelines on how a worker's ability to perform the work demands should be measured.[46–49] The U.S. Equal Employment Opportunity Commission provides guidelines on how to determine the content or criterion validities relating measurements to a job, but does not offer guidance as to what measurements should be taken and the method for how they are obtained.[50–53] Therefore, the medical expert must be cognizant of nuances of the different FCEs' content and protocols.

STRENGTH MEASUREMENTS

Although there is variability in content and methodologies among the different commercial and independent FCEs, determining strength is common to many physical functional assessment systems. Strength measurements are used to estimate the worker's physical capacity to determine if the worker possesses the necessary physical abilities required in manual material handling tasks.[54–58]

Strength is measured in terms of static (isometric) strength and/or dynamic strength. Static strength does not involve motion and is reflective of the ability to exert maximum force. Dynamic strength is measured as either isoinertial strength or as isokinetic strength. Static or dynamic strength measurements should be reflective of the nature of the work activity to which the worker is to be returned. If the activity primarily involves static actions, such as seen with stabilizing a structure or holding an object, it is more appropriate to measure static strength.[59] If the activity requires movement, dynamic strength is more appropriate.

Isometric Strength Testing

Isometric muscular contraction is the prolonged contraction of a muscle without a change in its length.[60,61] Characteristic of isometric strength is the application of force generated from voluntary isometric muscle contraction without resulting movement.[59]

Isometric strength measuring devices used in employment testing are standardized, but generally consist of an analog or digital force gauge and a restraint system to isolate muscle groups and limit body motion. Isometric forces measured using force transducers attached to a recording device can graphically present force-time measurements (**Fig. 4**).

There is controversy among researchers that static strength measurements are not reflective of real-world work activities, because, in most circumstances, people are moving because of the dynamic component of work.[59] However, others uphold the position that muscle contraction is need to initiate the "mass moment of inertia" (Newton's Second Law of Motion) required to change the object's state of motion.[62] Regardless of the controversy, isometric strength measurements are commonly assessed in employment situations.

Isometric strength measurements have been shown as predictors for risk of future injuries if the isometric strength measurements replicate specific material handling

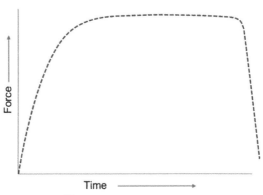

Fig. 4. Isometric force-time profile.

demands.[63–66] The direction and geometry of force application should closely simulate what is required of the activity. Body posture or limb position should simulate the work positions as closely as possible when isometric strength is measured.

FCEs report isometric strength measurements in terms of push/pull forces expressed as pounds or kilograms. Forces are generally applied vertically (to simulate lifting) or horizontally (to simulate pushing or pulling). It is difficult to categorize workers in DOT physical work demand levels using isometric force measurements because these measurements are not equated to weights or displacement. However, if the measurement has been demonstrated to replicate the actual material handling activity, inference can be made for the DOT physical work demand. If force-time profiles are used, inferences can also be made for O*NET descriptors for explosive strength (illustrated by the initial slope of time-force profile in **Fig. 4**) and static strength (illustrated by the plateau peak force in **Fig. 4**).

Isoinertial Strength

Isoinertial muscular contraction occurs when muscles contract against a load, resulting in motion. Characteristic of isoinertial strength measurement is that the mass of the object remains constant while muscle length changes with motion.[67,68] Muscle contraction changes with the speed of motion.[61] In a material handling setting, isoinertial strength represents muscle strength used for the dynamic material handling activities (eg, lifting, carrying, pushing, or pulling).

Two commonly used isoinertial protocols are the LIFTTEST and progressive isoinertial lift evaluation (PILE). The LIFTTEST uses a modified weight lifting device (similar to cable machines used for body building), in which the subject lifts and lowers stacked weights over a predetermined distance.[69,70] Using the PILE protocol, the subject progressively lifts and lowers incrementally increasing weights to the point of fatigue.[71,72]

Psychophysical factors can affect isoinertial strength measurements.[73–75] Psychophysical strength is a reflection of an individual's perception of what they can do (ie, what an individual subjectively believes they are capable of exerting).[74,76] The perceived strength may not be reflective of the person's maximum capacity due to voluntary or subconsciously imposed limitation. To account for psychophysical factors, Kroemer[67] and McDaniel[77] developed the Maximal Isoinertial Strength Test (MIST) protocol, in which the subject, not the evaluator, increases or decreases weight to their perceived acceptable level. Subjects determining their tolerance to specific activities has been demonstrated to be a factor in reducing risk for injures for work requiring exertions greater than the individual's voluntary (or perceived) strength.[65,78] Psychophysical strength assessments play a greater value in the ergonometric design of a job task rather than determining a worker's capacity to work.[79]

FCEs assessing isoinertial strength report measurements in terms of weights lifted or carried and how they are displaced (ie, vertical or horizontal distances). Vertical distances are expressed in anthropometric terms (eg, from floor to knuckle or waist height, knuckle or waist height to shoulder height, and above shoulder or overhead heights) or in terms of heights reflective of the work environment. Although horizontal distances are measured for carrying, the duration to complete this activity is rarely reported. Isoinertial lifting tests are shown to be predictive of a worker's ability for dynamic industrial lifting and carrying tasks if they closely simulate the essential functions of the work.[80] However, they have not been shown predictive of future injury.[81–83]

Isoinertial tests are more representative of real-world dynamic activities. Inferences can be made to the dynamic nature of lifting and carrying functions defined in DOT. Whole body movement during isoinertial tests allows the evaluator to offer observation-based inferences regarding postural requirements defined in DOT (see **Table 1**) and flexibility, coordination, and equilibrium descriptors in O*NET (see **Tables 3** and **4**).

Owing to the widespread use of DOT's physical work demands work levels (see **Fig. 1**), many FCE evaluators attempt to project the frequency of a strength measurement to classify the individual's capacity into one of these levels. However, there is no standard approach for how frequency is determined. In addition, inferences from isoinertial strength protocols, such as LIFTTEST, PILE, or MIST, have been used to estimate endurance and activity tolerances because lifting is repeated using progressively increasing weights. As with determining frequency, caution is advised when considering these inferences on endurance and activity tolerances in the absence of peer-reviewed studies.

Isokinetic Strength

Isokinetic muscular contractions occur when a muscle changes lengths to exert a constant force.[84] Characteristic of isometric strength measurement is controlling motion speed by varying the resistance to the movement.[85,86] In isokinetic strength assessments, the kinetic energy and velocity remain constant. Therefore, the mass (or resistance) must change. If the movement is too slow, resistance is decreased to allow the speed to increase. If the movement is too fast, the resistance is increased to slow its speed.

Most isokinetic strength measurement devices consist of a computer-controlled dynamometer and a restraining system to isolate a body segment (eg, ankle, knee, shoulder). The shaft of the dynamometer is attached to a cable system or lever apparatus and the shaft rotational controlled by increasing or decreasing resistance. To maintain a fixed speed and constant kinetic energy, resistance is increased or decreased by controlling the shaft's rotation speed. The resistance an individual encounters depends on their effort. If the speed is too fast, the resistance is increased. If the speed is too slow, the resistance is decreased.

Measurements are provided in terms of torque forces, power (watts) and rate of angular displacement (ie, degrees/s). Isokinetic measurements are not reflective of either DOT or O*NET function descriptors. Applicability of isokinetic strength measurements to determine ability to perform material handing work activities is questioned[87,88] because of the difficulty relating to real-world industrial settings, in which the mass properties of objects do not change during material handling.

USING FUNCTIONAL CAPACITY EVALUATION STRENGTH MEASUREMENTS TO DETERMINE A WORKER'S ABILITY TO RETURN TO WORK

There are no comprehensive peer review studies demonstrating that FCEs are predictive of future injuries used for RTW evaluations.[82] However, inferences can be made from peer-reviewed studies where work-specific FCEs (ie, simulating the essential function of the job), used in the pre-placement or pre-employment process, reduced the incidence of work of future injuries.[89–93] Work-related isometric strength measurements have been shown as predictors for risk of future injuries if the measurements are closely matched to the specific material handling demands.[63,64] Workers exceeding their physicophysical strength capabilities determined when isoinertial strength have been demonstrated to have less prevalent low back injuries[94,95] Isokinetic strength measurements are poor predictors for back injuries.[96]

USING FUNCTIONAL CAPACITY EVALUATIONS IN FORMULATION OF MEDICAL EXPERT OPINIONS

A common question asked of FCEs is "Is the FCE valid?" In the context of FCEs, validity refers how correctly FCEs reflects an individual's ability to perform a task or the job. Although this question is often asked of medicolegal experts, it is also applicable to the medical providers responsible for the employment medial determinations for RTW and FFD determinations. The question cannot be answered with a simple "yes" or "no" and requires examining an FCE's validity at several levels: FCE content, validity of the effort, and validity of the measurements (**Fig. 5**).

Functional Capacity Evaluation Content

FCE components must be representative of what is required of the job or task, that is, content validity. For example, an FCE assessing only lifting capacity is not considered reflective of jobs requiring carrying. If the job requires multiple tasks such as reaching, standing, climbing, and so forth, FCE measurements should address the corresponding tasks. Biomechanically, the FCE should simulate body positions and motion similar to those used on the job or for the task.

In most cases, it is not practical for an FCE to simulate every work activity required of a job. Therefore, many FCEs logically infer that, if an individual is capable of

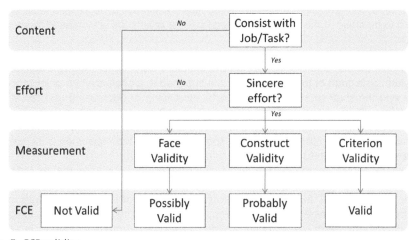

Fig. 5. FCE validity.

performing a more strenuous critical element of the job, the individual is logically capable of a lesser strenuous or critical components of the job. For example, if an individual demonstrates the capacity handing a variety of materials weight 50 pounds, it is assumed that the individual has the capacity to lift and/or carry less than 50 pounds.

Validity of Effort

The validity or sincerity of the effort is often mistakenly considered in the context of "malingering." Caution should be exercised with this perception because FCE's were not designed to determine an individual's integrity. It is not the intent of FCEs to function to detect "fakers" or "malingerers." However, the validity or sincerity of the effort is important when determining the reliability of the measurement.

FCEs incorporate many strategies to determine effort validity or sincerity.[97,98] Two popular strategies are to correlate *intra*-test physiologic responses (heart rate, blood pressure, perspirations) to the level of effort required of the task and/or use coefficients of variation (COV) limits. Although it is expected that physiologic responses change with more strenuous effort, it must be kept in mind that these responses are also affected by other factors such as physical conditioning, underlying cardiovascular conditions, medications, and so forth. COV is used to address the amount of variability between measurements.[99] Although some FCEs establish 15% COV limit,[100] caution should be exercised because this limit is arbitrary and other factors such as fatigue or an underlying impairment that can affect the reliability; multiple measurements can contribute to a high COV. As with using physiologic responses, caution is advised if this is a sole criteria to determine the sincerity of the effort.

Although physiologic responses and COV alone or in combination may not be strong indicators of the effort validity or sincerity, both can be augmented with *inter*-test behavioral and functional observations. Exaggerated symptoms complaints or inconsistent symptoms complaints with analogous maneuvers used in different tasks (eg, knee flexion is required for climbing upstairs or ladder, when squatting, or when lifting object from floor level) are useful clues to help determine effort validity. Similarly, premature termination of a task or inconsistent termination of task requiring analogous body positions/movements may provide useful information adding further insight to effort. Finally, correlating impact of an underlying impairment on the corresponding symptom complaint or termination of the test to provide plausible information regarding the sincerity of the effort. For example, it is not biologically palpable that a cervical impairment will result in low back pain when gait is assessed.

Validity of the Measurements

Three types of measurement validity should be considered when FCE results are reviewed: face validity, construct validity, and criterion validly. Face validity is the weakest type of validity, whereas criterion validity is the strongest type of validity.

In face validity, or at first glance "on the face of it," the measurement seems to be a representative of the construct. For example, FCEs measuring isometric strength are theoretically reflective of dynamic lifting, pushing, or pulling activities. In another example, FCEs using isokinetic testing to assess upper extremity isokinetic strength is in theory reflective of the ability to lift, carry, push, or pull.

Construct validity refers to the relationship of a measurement (or observation) to reality. The FCE constructs (ie, measurements) generalizes that an measurement measures what it purports to measure and closely reflects what is required of the job or the task. If the job or task is lifting, the FCE construct measures lifting. Isoinertial testing protocols, such as the PILE or LIFTTEST are considered content valid tests for lifting for jobs or tasks requiring lifting.

Criterion validity is similar to construct validity and represents the extent to which a measure is related to a specific outcome. If a task requirement is to lift a 35-pound box from a height of 15 to 40 inches and the individual demonstrates the ability to do so, the criteria is met. Similarly, if multiple tasks, with their unique criteria, are required of a job, those are the criteria that must be fulfilled.

Closely aligned to FCE measurement validity is measurement reliability. Reliability refers to the extent measurements are consistent. To assure reliable measurements, FCEs should repeat the measurement more than once. Reliability and validity are independent of each other. A measurement may be valid, but not reliable. Or the measurement may be reliable, but not valid. For example, isoinertial lifting is a valid method to assess a job where lifting is required. However, if repetitive measurements are not consistent, the measurement is not valid. Similarly, if the individual constantly replicates the isoinertial force on multiple exertions on a lift test, but the construct is for carrying, the pertinence of the measurement is questioned.

Predictive Validity

A corollary question to whether an FCE is valid is whether it is predictive of an injury. Predictive validity is a type of criterion validity correlating the test with concrete outcomes; does the test accurately predict what it is supposed to predict? FCEs have been demonstrated to be predictive of an individual's ability to work at jobs or perform certain task. When a workers' capacity is matched to a job requiring similar capacities, studies have demonstrated a decrease in the incidents of work-related injuries.[91] However, FCEs have not been demonstrated to predict whether or not injuries would occur.

SUMMARY

It is beneficial for both the worker and employer for the worker to return to work early as possible after an illness, injury, or prolonged absence. Because employers are ultimately responsible for the return to work decision, a medical RTW assessment is commonly required to assure that the worker is medically able to and physically capable of performing the job tasks. Consequently, many employers depend on the opinions from medical providers.

Valid FCEs can provide objective measurements of work-related strength capabilities and are useful in supporting a medical provider's opinion of a worker's ability to RTW or FFD. When using FCEs to formulate an opinion if a worker can return to work, the medical provider must consider if the measurement method simulates the actual work to which the individual is being returned. If FCE measurements simulate the characteristic of a material handling task, they can be predictive of the worker's physical abilities to return to work.

A valid FCE generally results in 1 of 2 outcomes: (1) demonstration that the worker is capable of the work task or (2) worker does not have the physical capability to perform the task or does not meet the work criteria. It is the responsibility of the medical provider to assure that there are no medical restrictions due to a health condition, even though the worker demonstrated sufficient physical capacity to perform the necessary tasks. If the worker does not have the capacity to perform the task, the medical provider should correlate the deficiency with a medical explanation of the impairment and can offer recommendations for accommodations.

REFERENCES

1. American College of Occupational and Environmental Medicine Stay-at-Work and Return-to-Work Process Improvement Committee. Preventing needless

work disability by helping people stay employed. J Occup Environ Med 2006; 48(9):972–87.

2. Howard KJ, Mayer TG, Gatchel RJ. Effects of Presenteeism in chronic occupational musculoskeletal disorders: stay at work is validated. J Occup Environ Med 2009;51(6):724–31.

3. Jurisic M, Bean M, Harbaugh J, et al. The personal physician's role in helping patients with medical conditions stays at work or return to work. J Occup Environ Med 2017;59(6):125–31.

4. Bureau of Labor Statistic, US Department of Labor. Employer-reported workplace injuries and illnesses – 2016. USDL-17-1482. Available at: https://www. bls.gov/news.release/osh.toc.htm. Accessed May 22, 2018.

5. Melton L, Anfield R, Kane G, et al. Reducing the incidence of short-term disability: testing the effectiveness of an absence prediction and prevention intervention using an experimental design. J Occup Environ Med 2012;54(12): 1441–6.

6. van Duijn M, Eijkemans MJ, Koes BW, et al. The effects of timing on the cost-effectiveness of interventions for workers on sick leave due to low back pain. J Occup Environ Med 2010;67:744–50.

7. Bardos, M, Burak H, Ben-Shalom, Y. Assessing the costs and benefits of return-to-work programs. 2015; Submitted to: U.S. Department of Labor Office of Disability Employment Policy 200 Constitution Avenue, NW Washington, DC 2010 Project Officer: Department of Labor contracted study/white paper: Meredith DeDona Contract Number: GS10F0050L/DOLQ121A21886/DOLU139435199.

8. Melhorn JM. Occupational orthopaedics in this millennium. Clin Orthop Relat Res 2001 Apr;(385):23–35.

9. Bednar JM, Baesher-Griffith P, Osterman AL. Worker compensation effect of state law on treatment cost and work status. Clin Orthop 1998;351:74–7.

10. Cocchiarella L, Anderson GBJ, editors. Guides to the evaluation of permanent impairment. 5th edition. AMA Press; 2001. p. 8.

11. Rondinelli RD, Duncan PW. The concepts of impairment and disability. In: Rondielli RD, Katz RT, editors. Impairment rating and disability evaluation. Philadelphia: WB Saunders; 2000. p. 19.

12. Thompson A, Bain D, Theriault ME. Pre-post evaluation of an integrated return to work planning program in workers' compensation assessment clinics. J Occup Environ Med 2017;58(2):215–8.

13. Christian JH. Physician role change in managed care: a frontline report. Occup Med 1998;13:851–69.

14. Baron S, Filios MS, Marovich SJ. Recognition of the relationship between patients' work and health: a qualitative evaluation of the need for clinical decision support (CDS) for worker health in five primary care practices. J Occup Environ Med 2017;59(11):245–50.

15. Merill RN, Pransky G, Hathaway J, et al. Illness and the workplace. A study of physicians and employers. J Fam Pract 1990;31:55–9.

16. Arif J, Pransky G, Fish J, et al. Return-to-work within a complex and dynamic organizational work disability system. J Occup Rehabil 2016;26:276–85.

17. Yassi A, Hassard TH, Kopoelow MM, et al. Evaluating medical performance in the diagnosis and treatment of occupational health problems: a standardized patient approach. J Occup Med 1990;32:582–5.

18. O'Fallon E, Hillson S. Brief report: physician discomfort and variability with disability assessments. J Gen Intern Med 2005;20:852–4.

19. Sokas RK, Kolb LS, Welch LS, et al. A single-session exercise to address medical residents' attitudes toward work disability evaluations. Acad Med 1995; 70:167.

20. Hanman B. Physical capacities and job placement. 1st edition. Stockholm (Sweden): Nordisk Rotogravyr; 1951. p. 79.

21. Anema JR, Van Der Giezen Am, Buijs PC, et al. Ineffective disability management by doctors is an obstacle for return to work: a cohort study on low back pain patients' sicklisted for 3-4 months. Occup Environ Med 2002;59:729–33.

22. Bono de AM. Communication between an occupational physician and other medical practitioners—an audit. Occup Med 1997;47:349–56.

23. United States Department of Labor. Selected characteristics of occupations defined in the revised dictionary of occupational titles. Washington, DC: U.S. Department of Labor Employment and Training Administration; 1993. U.S. Government Printing Office Superintendent of Documents. Mail Stop: SSOP, 20402-9328.

24. Physical exertion requirements, 20 C.F.R. §404.1567.

25. Dictionary of Occupational Titiles Appendix C. Components of the definition trailer. Available at: https://occupationalinfo.org/appendxc_1.html. Accessed March 14, 2017.

26. 20 CFR § 404.1567 Physical exertion requirements.

27. United States Department of Labor. Selected characteristics of occupations defined in the revised dictionary of occupational titles. Revised 4th Edition Appendix C Physical Demands, op. cit. 1993;C1-C4. Washington, DC: U.S. Department of Labor Employment and Training Administration; 1993. U.S. Government Printing Office Superintendent of Documents. Mail Stop: SSOP, 20402-9328.

28. United States Department of Labor. Selected characteristics of occupations defined in the revised dictionary of occupational titles. Revised 4th Edition Appendix C Physical Demands, op. cit. 1993;C1-C4. Washington, DC: Department of Labor Employment and Training Administration; 1993. U.S. Government Printing Office Superintendent of Documents. Mail Stop: SSOP, 20402-9328.

29. U.S. Department of Labor, Herman AM, Abraham KG. Revising the standard occupational classification system. 1999; Report 929. Available at: www.bls.gov/soc/socrpt929.pdf. Accessed August 21, 2017.

30. Mariani M. Replace with a database: O*NET replaces the Dictionary of Occupational Titles, occupational outlook quarterly 1999. Available at: www.bls.gov/careeroutlook/1999/Spring/art01.pdf. Accessed June 1, 2017.

31. Soo Hoo ER. Social security disability and the AMA guides. AMA Guides Newsletter 2015;5–10.

32. O*NET Resource Center. Available at: www.onetcenter.org/. Accessed April 19, 2018.

33. About O*NET. Available at: https://www.onetcenter.org/overview.html. Accessed June 20, 2018.

34. Herman AM, Abraham KG. Revising the Standard Occupational Classification System June 1999:Report 929. Available at: www.bls.gov/soc/socrpt929.pdf. Accessed February 3, 2018.

35. The O*NET Content Model. Available at: www.onetcenter.org/content.html. Accessed April 19, 2018.

36. Occupational Information Network (O*NET). Available at: www.doleta.gov/programs/onet/. Accessed January 21, 2016.

37. Available at: www.onetonline.org/find/descriptor/browse/Abilities/1.A.3/. Accessed February 3, 2018.
38. O*NET OnLine Help. Available at: www.onetonline.org/help/online/scales/. Accessed February 3, 2018.
39. Noone JH, Bohle P, Mackey M. Matching work capacity and job demands: toward an enhanced measure of work ability. J Occup Environ Med 2015; 57(12):1360–4.
40. Pransky GS, Dempsey PG. Practical aspect of functional capacity evaluations. J Occup Rehabil 2004;14:217–29.
41. Strong S, Paptiste S, Clark J, et al. Use of functional capacity evaluation in workplaces and the compensation system: a report on workers' and users' perceptions. Work 2004;23:67–77.
42. Matheson L. The functional capacity evaluation. In: Anderson G, Demeter S, Smith G, editors. Disability evaluations. 2nd edition. Chicago: Mosby Yearbook; 2003. p. 748–68.
43. King PM, Tuckwell N, Barret TE. A critical review of functional capacity evaluations. Phys Ther 1988;78(8):852–66.
44. Rucker KS, Wehman P, Kregel J. Analysis of functional assessment instruments for disability/rehabilitation programs. US Social Security Administration contracted study/white paper: SSA Contract No. 600-95-21914.
45. Matheson LN, Kaskutas V, McCowan S, et al. Development of a database of functional assessment measures related to work disability. J Occup Rehabil 2001;11:177.
46. American Physical Therapy Association. Orthopedic Section. Occupational Health Physical Therapy: Evaluating functional capacity guidelines. Rescinded as APTA guidelines in May 2011, adopted by Orthopaedic Section BOD July 11, 2011. Available at: https://www.apta.org/uploadedFiles/APTAorg/About_Us/Policies/BOD/Practice/CriteriaforStandardsofPractice.pdf. Accessed May 20, 2018.
47. Guide to physical therapist practice. Available at: http://guidetoptpractice.apta.org/. Accessed May 20, 2018.
48. American Occupational Therapy Association. Functional capacity evaluations. Available at: https://www.aota.org/About-Occupational-Therapy/Professionals/WI/Capacity-Eval.aspx. Accessed May 24, 2018.
49. Rothstein JM, Campbell SK, Echternach JL, et al. Standards for tests and measurements in physical therapy practice. Phys Ther 1991;71(8):589–622.
50. United States Equal Employment Opportunity Commission. 29 CFR Ch. XIV, Part 1607 – uniform guidelines on employee selection procedures. Washington, D.C: U.S. Government Printing Office; 1991. p. 1991.
51. United States Equal Employment Opportunity Commission. A technical assistance manual on the employment provisions (Title I) of the Americans with disabilities Act. Washington, DC: U.S. Government Printing Office; 1992.
52. United States Equal Employment Opportunity Commission. ADA technical assistance manual addendum. Available at: www.eeoc.gov/policy/docs/adamanual_add.html. Accessed June 1, 2018.
53. Soo Hoo ER, Demeter SL. Job validation studies and physical agility testing: is the vendor telling you what they think you want or are you telling them what you need? AMA Guides Newsletter 2016;5–10.
54. Gallagher S, Moore JS, Stobbe TJ. Physical strength assessment in ergonomics. American Industrial Hygiene Association. Fairfax (VA): AIHA Press; 1998.

55. Chaffin DB, Anderson GBJ. Occupational biomechanics. 3rd edition. New York: John Wiley & Sons; 1999. p. 501–23.
56. Gallagher S, Moore JS, Stobbe TJ. Physical strength assessment in ergonomics. American Industrial Hygiene Association, AIHA Press; pp. 7–9.
57. King PM, Tuckwell N, Barret TE. A critical review of functional capacity evaluations. Phys Ther 1988;78(8):852–66.
58. Menard MR, Hoens AM. Objective evaluation of functional capacity: medial, occupational, and legal settings. J Orthop Sports Phys Ther 1994;19:249–60.
59. Gallagher S, Moore JS, Stobbe TJ. Physical strength assessment in ergonomics. American Industrial Hygiene Association, AIHA Press; p. 11.
60. Gallagher S, Moore JS, Stobbe TJ. Physical strength assessment in ergonomics. American Industrial Hygiene Association, AIHA Press; pp. 11–20.
61. Chaffin DB, Anderson GBJ, Martin BJ. Occupational biomechanics. 3nd edition. New York: John Wiley & Sons; 1999. p. 37–8.
62. Özkaya N, Nordin M. Fundamentals of biomechanics equilibrium, motion and deformation. 2nd edition. New York: Springer Science + Business Medical, Inc.; 1999. p. 47–80.
63. Troup JD, Martin JW, Lloyd DC. Back pain in industry. A prospective study. Spine 1981;6:61–9.
64. Battie MC, Bigos SJ, Fisher LD, et al. Isometric lift strength as a predictor of industrial back pain. Spine 1989;14:851–6.
65. Chaffin DB, Herrin GD, Keyserling VM. Pre-employment strength testing: an updated position. J Occup Med 1978;20(6):403–8.
66. Keyserling VW, Herrin GD, Chaffin DB. Isometric strength testing as a means of controlling medical incidents on strenuous jobs. J Occup Med 1980;22(5): 322–36.
67. Kroemer KHE. Development of LIFTEST: a dynamic technique to assess the induvial capacity to lift material, final report. 1982;NIOSH contracted report/white paper: Contract 210-79-0041.
68. Kroemer KHE, Marras WS, McGlothlin DR, et al. On the measurement of human strength. Int J Ind Ergon 1990;6:199–210.
69. Kroemer KHE. Development of LIFTEST: a dynamic technique to assess the induvial capacity to lift material, final report. 1982;NIOSH Contract 210-79-0041.
70. McDaniel JW, Shandis RJ, Madole SW. Weight lifting capabilities of air force basic trainees (AFAMRL-TR-0001). Dayton, OH: Wright Patterson AFBDH. Air Force AerospaceMedical Research Laboratory; 1983.
71. Mayer TG, Barnes D, Kishino ND, et al. Progressive isoinertial lifting equation – I.A. standardized protocol and normative database. Spine 1988;13(8):993–7.
72. Mayer TG, Barnes D, Nicholas G, et al. Progressive isoinertial lifting equation II. A comparison with isokinetic lifting in a chronic low back pain industrial population. Spine 1988;13(8):998–1002.
73. Ayoub MM, Mita A. Manual material handling. London: Taylor and Francis; 1989. p. 241–2.
74. Chaffin DB, Anderson GBJ, Martin BJ. Occupational biomechanics. 3rd edition. New York: John Wiley & Sons; 1999. p. 101–2.
75. Gibson L, Strong J. A review of functional capacity evaluation practice. Work 1997;9(3):3–11.
76. Matheson LN, Mooney v, Grant JE, et al. A test to measure lift capacity of physically impaired adults, part 1 – development and reliability testing. Spine 1995; 20919:2119–29.

77. McDaniel JW, Shandis RJ, Madole SW. Weight lifting capabilities of air force basic trainees (AFAMRL-TR-0001). Wright Patterson AFBDH, Air Force Aerospace Medical Research Laboratory; 1983.
78. Keyserling WM, Herrin GD, Chaffin DB, et al. Establishing an industrial strength testing program. Am Ind Hyg Assoc J 1980;41:730–6.
79. Snook SH. Approaches to control of back pain in industry: job design, job placement, and education/training. Occup Med 1987;2:45–59.
80. Chaffin DB, Anderson GBJ, Martin BJ. Occupational biomechanics. 3nd edition. New York: John Wiley & Sons; 1999. p. 108–19.
81. Gallagher S, Moore JS, Stobbe TJ. Physical strength assessment in ergonomics. American Industrial Hygiene Association, AIHA Press; p 31.
82. Chaffin DB, Anderson GBJ, Martin BJ. Occupational biomechanics. 3nd edition. New York: John Wiley & Sons; 1999. p. 501–23.
83. Stevenson JM, Greenhourn DR, Bryan JT, et al. Gender differences in performance of a selection test using the incremental lifting machine. Appl Ergon 1996;27(1):45–52.
84. Hilslop H, Perrine JJ. The isokinetic concept of exercise. Phys Ther 1967;47: 114–7.
85. Newton M, Waddell G. Trunk strength testing with iso-machines. Spine 1993;18: 801–11.
86. Newton M, Thow M, Somerville D, et al. Trunk strength testing with iso-machines. Part 2: experimental evaluation of the cybex II back testing system in normal subjects and patients with chronic low back pain. Spine 1993;18(7):812–24.
87. Gallagher S, Moore JS, Stobbe TJ. Physical strength assessment in ergonomics. American Industrial Hygiene Association, AIHA Press; p 53.
88. Dueker JA, Ritchie SM, Knox TJ, et al. Isokinetic trunk testing and employment. J Occup Med 1994;36(1):42–8.
89. Biering-Sorensen F. Physical measurements as risk indicators for low back trouble over a one-year period. Spine 1984;9:106–19.
90. Rayson MP. Fitness for work: the need for conducting a job analyses. Occup Med 2000;50(6):434–6.
91. Harbin G, Olson J. Post-offer, pre-placement testing in industry. Am J Ind Med 2005;47:296–307.
92. Keyserling WM, Herrin GD, Chaffin DB, et al. Establishing an industrial strength testing program. Am Ind Hyg Assoc J 1980;41:730–6.
93. Toeppen-Sprigg B. Importance of job analysis with functional capacity matching in medical case management: a physician's perspective. Work 2000;15(2):133–7.
94. Chaffin DB, Anderson GBJ, Martin BJ. Occupational biomechanics. 3nd edition. New York: John Wiley & Sons; 1999. p. 94.
95. Snook SH. The design of manual handling task. Ergonomics 1978;21(12): 963–85.
96. Mostardi RA, Noe DA, Kovacik MW, et al. Isokinetic Lifting strength and occupational injury: a prospective study. Spine 1992;17(2):189–93.
97. Lechner D, Bradbury S, Bradley L. Detecting sincerity of effort: a summary of methods and approaches. Phys Ther 1998;78(8):867–88.
98. Matheson L. How do you know that he tried his best? Reliability crisis in industrial rehabilitation. Industrial Rehabilitation Quarterly 1988;1(1):11–2.
99. Zar J. Biostatistical analysis. 5th.edition. Upper Saddle River (NJ): Prentice-Hall, Inc.; 2007. ISBN:0131008463 Englewood Cliffs, NJ: Prentice-Hall, Inc.
100. Klimek E, Strait J. Volition in impairment rating: the validity of effort assessment. J Occup Med 1997;6(2):9–18.

The Work Disability Functional Assessment Battery (WD-FAB)

Alan M. Jette, PT, PhD[a,b,*], Pengsheng Ni, MD, MPH[c],
Elizabeth Rasch, PT, PhD[d], Elizabeth Marfeo, PhD, MPH, OTR/L[e],
Christine McDonough, PT, PhD[f], Diane Brandt, PT, PhD[g],
Lewis Kazis, ScD[h], Leighton Chan, MD, MPH[i]

KEYWORDS

- Rehabilitation • Health policy • Quality of life • Outcomes

KEY POINTS

- In the United States, national disability programs are challenged to adjudicate millions of work disability claims each year in a timely and accurate manner.
- The Work Disability Functional Assessment Battery (WD-FAB) was developed to provide work disability agencies and other interested parties a comprehensive and efficient approach to profiling a person's function related to their ability to work.
- The WD-FAB is constructed using contemporary item response theory methods to yield an instrument that can be administered efficiently using computerized adaptive testing techniques.
- The WD-FAB could provide relevant information about work-related functioning for a wide range of clinical and policy applications.

Disclosure: The development of the manuscript was supported, in part, by SSA Contracts HHSN269201200005C and HHSN269201200009I.
 a Boston University Sargent College of Health and Rehabilitation Sciences, Boston, MA, USA; b MGH Institute of Health Professions, Charlestown Navy Yard, 36 1st Avenue, Boston, MA 02129-4557, USA; c Department of Health Law, Policy and Management, BU School of Public Health, 715 Albany Street T5W, Boston, MA 02118, USA; d Epidemiology and Biostatistics Section, Rehabilitation Medicine Department, National Institutes of Health, Mark O. Hatfield Clinical Research Center, 6707 Democracy Boulevard, Suite 856, MSC 5493, Bethesda, MD 20892-5493, USA; e Department of Occupational Therapy, Tufts University, Health & Productive Aging Lab (HPAL), 574 Boston Avenue, Suite 216G, Medford, MA 02155, USA; f School of Health and Rehabilitation Sciences, University of Pittsburgh, Bridgeside Point I, 100 Technology Drive, Pittsburgh, PA 15219, USA; g Social Security Advisory Board, 400 Virginia Avenue Southwest, Suite 625, Washington, DC 20024, USA; h Health Outcomes Unit and Center for the Assessment of Pharmaceutical Practices (CAPP) (Est. 2000), Boston University School of Public Health, 715 Albany Street, Talbot 5 West (532), Boston, MA 02118, USA; i Rehabilitation Medicine Department, Clinical Center, National Institutes of Health, Building 10, Room 1-1469 10 Center Drive, MSC 1604, Bethesda, MD 20892-1604, USA
* Corresponding author. MGH Institute of Health Professions, Charlestown Navy Yard, 36 1st Avenue, Boston, MA 02129-4557, USA.
E-mail address: alanmjette@gmail.com

Phys Med Rehabil Clin N Am 30 (2019) 561–572
https://doi.org/10.1016/j.pmr.2019.03.004
1047-9651/19/© 2019 Elsevier Inc. All rights reserved.

INTRODUCTION

Work disability is a major public health problem that is associated with poverty, lack of access to health care, and limitations in other important aspects of social participation.[1,2] Historically, many work disability evaluation processes, including the US Social Security Administration's (SSA) disability determination process, focused on an individual's symptoms or impairments. However, the relationship between symptoms and work performance is not always clear, and the weak relationship between them has been increasingly recognized as one of the fundamental challenges in work disability assessment.[3] For example, someone who may display maladaptive behavior patterns may function well in a job that is relatively solitary and requires little interaction with others. Similarly, a person who has pain when standing or sitting for long periods may be able to function in a job that allows frequent rest breaks and periodic body position changes. These examples illustrate how work disability represents a multidimensional concept that goes beyond symptoms and impairments to include aspects of environment, functional abilities, and behaviors. Consequently, evaluating work capacity for people who demonstrate physical health or mental health problems proves difficult from impairment- or symptom-based perspectives alone.

APPLICATION OF THE INTERNATIONAL CLASSIFICATION OF FUNCTIONING, DISABILITY, AND HEALTH TO WORK DISABILITY ASSESSMENT

Current concepts of disability emphasize functional, behaviorally based definitions as they relate to factors in the work environment. To be more specific, work disability can be viewed as the outcome of the interaction between an individual's underlying capabilities in the context of the workplace environment.[4] This dynamic notion of disability has been most recently characterized in the World Health Organization's (WHO) International Classification of Functioning, Disability, and Health (ICF), which includes biologic, mental, personal, and social perspectives of disability.[5,6]

Factors associated with work disability are multifactorial and extend beyond individual symptoms and impairments indicative of the underlying and potential work-disability medical condition. In addition to the symptoms of a health condition, important factors to consider when assessing work ability include a person's cognitive status, education, age, underlying vocational skills, previous work, and the person-environment fit of the job demands.[7–10] For this article, the authors focus on a recent effort to improve person-level measures of an individual's functioning at the level of the person (as opposed to the cellular, organ, or organ system level) relevant to work. In developing this approach, the authors used the ICF as a conceptual foundation to organize and develop a content model for the Work Disability Functional Assessment Battery (WD-FAB), consisting of new measures of physical and mental health functioning.[11] By adding functional assessment items to the traditional impairment-based model, the WD-FAB attempts to provide a more comprehensive representation of a person's ability to work. In this article, the authors describe 3 stages of development and revision of the WD-FAB and discuss its usefulness in work disability evaluation.

CONCEPTUAL FRAMEWORK FOR THE WORK DISABILITY FUNCTIONAL ASSESSMENT BATTERY

To guide development of the WD-FAB items, content models were created to provide a comprehensive structure for development of an outcome measure of Physical Functioning and Mental Health relevant to work. The initial content model developed to guide construction of the WD-FAB Physical Function items is illustrated in **Fig. 1**

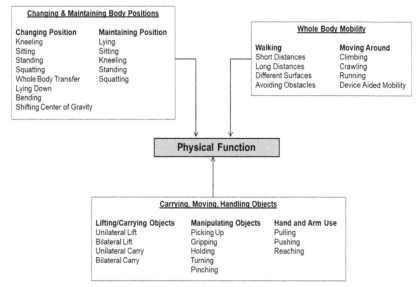

Fig. 1. Physical function content model.

and consists of 3 domains: (1) Changing and maintaining body position, (2) Whole body mobility, and (3) Carrying, moving, and handling objects, focused on the "activity" level of the ICF. These 3 major domains reflect integration of the ICF, existing work-related conceptual models, and current physical health outcome measurement instruments.[12,13]

Subdomains within the primary physical function domains include components such as maintaining and changing body position, gross motor body movements, postural control, and functional mobility that characterize various aspects of physical health applicable for assessing a person's overall potential ability to function in a work environment. By expanding traditional models of physical impairment, this content model provided an opportunity to build a comprehensive item pool of questions targeting overall physical functioning relevant to the context of work.

The WD-FAB Mental Health Function content model presented in **Fig. 2** suggests there are 5 major domains: (1) Behavior control, (2) Basic interactions, (3) Temperament and personality, (4) Adaptability, and (5) Workplace behaviors. These 5 key domains were developed based on the ICF, other selected models of work disability, and more theoretic literature discussing aspects of human behavior, personality, and social skills.[14,15]

Subdomains of the primary mental health concept represent individual components, such as mood and emotions, behavioral modulation adaptation, adaptability, temperament and personality, and interpersonal interaction skills that may act independently or interact to characterize mental health functioning. This integrated perspective provides a comprehensive structure upon which a final item pool of questions was built for the WD-FAB enabling assessment of a wide spectrum of mental health functioning skills.

Both the physical function and the mental health function content models guided the development of the WD-FAB, a self-reported measure of a person's traits, characteristics, and abilities related to successful functioning in a workplace environment.

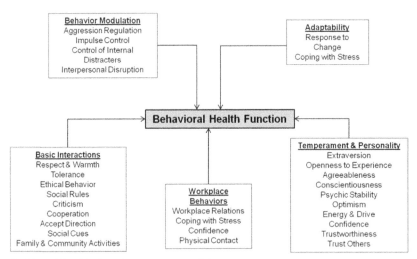

Fig. 2. Mental health function content model.

DEVELOPMENT OF WORK DISABILITY FUNCTIONAL ASSESSMENT BATTERY$_{1.0}$

In 2011, the WD-FAB$_{1.0}$ was created to allow the SSA to collect more systematic and comprehensive information about claimants' functioning. The first step was to develop a pool of questionnaire items to include in the WD-FAB and involved several sequential steps, which included a comprehensive literature review; gap analysis; item generation with expert panel input; stakeholder interviews; cognitive interview testing; and a cross-sectional survey administered by Internet and telephone surveys to a sample of 1017 SSA work disability claimants, and a normative sample of 999 adults from the US general population. Details on item development and surveys are available elsewhere.[11,12,14]

Analysis of the WD-FAB consisted of 2 steps. First, the factor structure of the item pool was examined using exploratory factor analyses, confirmatory factor analyses (CFA), and expert content review. In the second step, item response theory (IRT) methods were used to identify a comprehensive set of questions for the WD-FAB that defined each relevant construct included in the content models, in this case, physical function and mental health domains relevant to one's ability to work (see **Figs. 1** and **2**). IRT modeling was used to assess the fit items created and administered to the study samples to several hierarchical scales that arrayed items from low to high functioning within each scale. These methods were then used to assign, or calibrate, each item to a location on its appropriate WD-FAB scale based on the information it provided. Developing an instrument using IRT methods allows the user to determine scale score estimation from any subset of questions, because they are based on the calibrated item bank. In addition, computerized adaptive testing (CAT) administration methods could be used to administer the WD-FAB, allowing a computerized algorithm to tailor item selection in real time, selecting the item that will provide the most information at the respondent's estimated functional level.[16] CAT programs use a simple form of artificial intelligence that selects questions tailored to the test-taker and thereby shortens or lengthens the test to achieve the level of precision desired by a user. The combination of IRT and CAT methods allows the WD-FAB to generate highly precise scores with relatively low assessment burden.

WORK DISABILITY FUNCTIONAL ASSESSMENT BATTERY$_{1.0}$ RESULTS

The physical function item pool administered to the WD-FAB$_{1.0}$ samples consisted of 139 items. Initial factor analyses revealed a 4-factor solution, which allowed for separate characterization of physical functioning. Subsequent IRT analyses resulted in the 5 following unidimensional WD-FAB physical function scales, for a total of 102 items:

1. Changing and maintaining body position
2. Whole body mobility
3. Upper-body function
4. Upper-extremity fine motor
5. Wheelchair mobility

High CAT accuracy was demonstrated by strong correlations between simulated CAT scores and those from the full item banks.[13,17]

In the mental health domain, CFA specified that a 4-factor model characterizing a person's self-efficacy, mood and emotions, behavioral control, and social interactions had the optimal fit with the data and was also consistent with the authors' hypothesized content model for characterizing mental health functioning. Subsequent IRT analyses supported the unidimensionality of 4 WD-FAB$_{1.0}$ mental health function scales:

1. Mood and emotions
2. Self-efficacy
3. Social interactions
4. Behavioral control

All WD-FAB mental health scales demonstrated strong psychometric properties, including reliability, accuracy, and breadth of coverage. High correlations of the simulated 5- or 10-item CATs with the full item bank indicated robust ability of the CAT approach to comprehensively characterize mental health function along 4 distinct dimensions.[15,17,18]

The WD-FAB$_{1.0}$ instrument contributed important new methodology for measuring the physical function and mental health functioning of adults applying for work disability support. Initial testing and evaluation of the WD-FAB$_{1.0}$ demonstrated good accuracy, reliability, and content coverage along all 9 unidimensional scales.[17,18] Using the CAT-based approach to administer the WD-FAB$_{1.0}$ offers the ability to collect standardized, comprehensive functional information in an efficient way, which could prove useful in the context of evaluating applicants for work disability programs.

DEVELOPMENT OF WORK DISABILITY FUNCTIONAL ASSESSMENT BATTERY$_{2.0}$

One of the unique benefits of building the WD-FAB using IRT methods is that IRT-based instruments can be updated and expanded, or replenished, by adding new items and calibrating them onto the existing scoring metric,[19] which means that evidence of the measurement properties of the instrument would apply across different versions of an instrument.

Although WD-FAB$_{1.0}$ represented significant conceptual progress with functional items across a wide continuum with reasonable item density, there was a need to expand the WD-FAB to ensure it reflected comprehensive item content that was applicable for use among people with a wide range of physical and mental health conditions that might affect their ability to work. To conduct replenishment of WD-FAB$_{1.0}$, both new items and some existing items from WD-FAB$_{1.0}$ that served as anchors to the original item calibrations were used to calibrate and replenish the WD-FAB$_{1.0}$ scales. With this in mind, 2 replenishment studies were undertaken to build on the initial structure of the WD-FAB$_{1.0}$, adding content to current domains, which resulted in WD-FAB$_{2.0}$ and WD-FAB$_{3.0}$ instruments.

WORK DISABILITY FUNCTIONAL ASSESSMENT BATTERY$_{2.0}$

The initial WD-FAB$_{1.0}$ physical function domain developed in 2011 included 4 scales: Changing and maintaining body position, which includes the ability to assume, maintain, and transfer among various positions, such as lying, kneeling, sitting, squatting, and standing; Whole body mobility, which includes the ability to move around from 1 place to another, including crawling, walking, and running; Upper-body function, which entails reaching, lifting, pulling, pushing, and carrying; and Upper-extremity fine motor, which included manipulation of objects requiring dexterity. In developing WD-FAB$_{2.0}$, the authors expanded the breadth of content covered in the WD-FAB$_{1.0}$ physical function scales to add more difficult items in upper-extremity fine-motor function, easier items in upper-body function, to add more items to other scales and to provide new items addressing the subdomain of community mobility, which the authors defined as driving or using mass transportation to get around one's community. [20]

In the mental health domain, WD-FAB$_{1.0}$ characterized mental health function along the following domains: mood and emotions, social interactions, self-efficacy, and behavioral control.[21] Mood and emotions represented a range of a person's internal emotional state that can affect a person's ability to work and encompassed feelings such as depression and anxiety. Social interactions focused on a person's ability to interact with others. Self-efficacy represented a range of concepts, such as resilience, adaptability, trust, and motivation. Last, behavioral control captured traits such as emotional regulation and anger.

For replenishment of the WD-FAB$_{1.0}$ scales, the authors recruited content experts with expertise in measurement and treatment of physical function limitations and disability to help investigators expand content coverage of WD-FAB$_{1.0}$. The ICF was again used as the theoretic framework for replenishment of the WD-FAB$_{1.0}$ physical function and mental health.[5] Existing items were coded according to the ICF framework and hierarchically ordered using IRT calibration as in the initial field study.

Newly developed and anchor physical function questions from WD-FAB$_{1.0}$ were administered to a sample of 3532 recent SSA applicants for work disability benefits and a sample of 2025 adults representing working-age adults living in the United States.[20] In the mental health domain, new and a sample of existing WD-FAB$_{1.0}$ items were administered to a stratified sample of 1695 claimants applying for the SSA work disability benefits, and a general population sample of 2025 working-age adults.[21] Factor analyses and IRT methods were used to calibrate and link the new items to the existing WD-FAB$_{1.0}$ scales to create the WD-FAB$_{2.0}$ instrument. The authors conducted CAT simulations to examine the psychometric properties of WD-FAB$_{2.0}$.[20,21]

WORK DISABILITY FUNCTIONAL ASSESSMENT BATTERY$_{2.0}$ RESULTS

In the physical function domain, CFA and IRT analyses supported integration of 44 new items into 3 existing WD-FAB scales and the addition of a new 11-item scale (community mobility). The final physical function domain, consisting of basic mobility (56 items), upper-body function (34 items), fine-motor function (45 items), and community mobility (11 items), demonstrated acceptable psychometric properties.[20] In the mental health domain, factor and IRT analyses supported the inclusion of 4 subdomains: cognition and communication (68 items), self-regulation (34 items), resilience and sociability (29 items), and mood and emotions (34 items). All scales in $WD\text{-}FAB_{2.0}$ yielded acceptable psychometric properties. [21]

DEVELOPMENT OF WORK DISABILITY FUNCTIONAL ASSESSMENT BATTERY$_{3.0}$

The main purpose of creating $WD\text{-}FAB_{3.0}$ was to include new items that could be used to expand the breadth and depth of content covered in the previously developed WD-FAB versions. Because the WD-FAB has undergone replenishment in the past, the authors did not expect substantial gains in performance of the number of items administered in the CATs. Rather, they hoped to add items with content and clinical relevance that would expand content coverage across each content domain in the WD-FAB. Specifically, in the physical function domain, the authors aimed to include activity items specific to pain and fatigue. They expected the effects of pain and fatigue to be represented in responses to questions about "activities," and they included them because of their importance to work disability determination. The authors also addressed coverage of difficulty of different work roles (eg, sedentary, light, medium, heavy, and very heavy job classifications). In the mental health domain, they aimed to enhance resilience and sociability and self-regulation scales' breadth, depth, and reliability. They were able to add a total of 23 items (basic mobility, 7; upper-body function, 4; fine motor, 6; self-regulation, 1; resilience and sociability, 5 items) to the WD-FAB. Seven items in the physical function domain were added to address pain and fatigue.

The overall approach, as in developing $WD\text{-}FAB_{2.0}$, was to enlist content experts to assist in creating new items addressing the objectives and then to conduct a calibration field study. The authors selected content experts with knowledge in measurement and treatment of functional limitations and disability.

In developing $WD\text{-}FAB_{3.0}$, the authors administered a subset of existing items, called "anchor items," in conjunction with the new items to 2 samples to enable them to cocalibrate the new items onto the same existing scale. The analysis done in the SSA claimant sample was repeated in the general working-age sample to allow validation of factor structure and IRT analysis results. For the calibration field study, the final $WD\text{-}FAB_{3.0}$ instrument included the following number of new/anchor items, respectively: basic mobility, 11/10; upper-body function, 10/7; fine-motor function, 9/9; self-regulation, 10/7; resilience and sociability, 10/6.

For the calibration field study, the authors recruited 2 samples: 1051 recent SSA work disability claimants and a general working-age sample of 1000 US adults (aged 21–66 years). The surveys were administered via the Web or by telephone.

To analyze each scale, the authors examined the fit of all possible combinations of new items combined with anchor items using CFA. To select the final item set, the authors considered item fit and content relative to the authors' stated objectives.

CAT algorithms were created for each of the scales using weighted likelihood estimation to estimate the score and standard error. The algorithm was programmed to select the initial item at midlevel difficulty, calculate the score estimate, administer subsequent items with the optimal information yield for that score, and then recalculate the score based on the subsequent response. The stopping rule used in the algorithm required a minimum of 5 items, maximum of 10, and reliability ≥ 0.90. Summary scores were transformed to T scores with mean = 50, standard deviation = 10, with lower scores indicating lower function.

WORK DISABILITY FUNCTIONAL ASSESSMENT BATTERY$_{3.0}$ RESULTS

The authors' CFA results from $WD\text{-}FAB_{3.0}$ provided additional support for the factor structure of the WD-FAB. Their comparison of CFA results from $WD\text{-}FAB_{2.0}$ and

WD-FAB$_{3.0}$ revealed very similar fit from 2.0 to 3.0, with slightly to substantially improved fit for WD-FAB$_{3.0}$ compared with WD-FAB$_{2.0}$ in claimant data. All the model fit indices were in the acceptable range, so the factor structure held between the WD-FAB$_{2.0}$ and WD-FAB$_{3.0}$ general working-age adult samples. Simulation analyses showed that there were small gains in performance of the CAT. For example, fewer items were required for the resilience and sociability scale, and a decrease in percent at the ceiling was achieved for the fine-motor scale. Distributions of the claimant and working-age sample scores showed that there were no ceiling or floor effects for the claimant scores, and that scores for claimants, as expected, were lower than scores of the general working-age sample (**Fig. 3**). **Fig. 4** displays the domains of WD-FAB$_{3.0}$ along with the number of items in each domain item pool.

APPLICATIONS

The WD-FAB represents a significant psychometric and conceptual advancement in the area of assessment related to work in several ways. First, a unique feature of the WD-FAB is its conceptual foundation that uses principles outlined by the WHO's ICF classification. The ICF highlights the multifactorial nature of disability by focusing on biologic, mental, personal, and social perspectives of disability.[5] Factors related to a person's ability to work are complex and extend beyond disease symptoms and impairments alone, but include factors such as functional activity limitations, psychological well-being, and contextual factors. In developing both the physical and

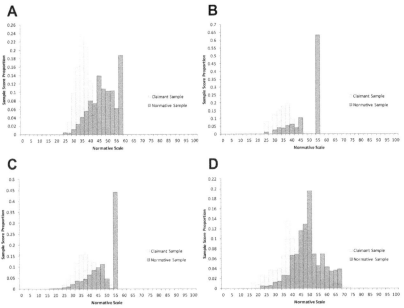

Fig. 3. (*A*) Basic mobility scale distribution in claimant and normative samples. (*B*) Upper-body function scale distribution in claimant and normative samples. (*C*) Fine-motor function scale distribution in claimant and normative samples. (*D*) Resilience and sociability scale distribution in claimant and normative samples. (*E*) Self-regulation scale distribution in claimant and normative samples. (*F*) Mood and emotion scale distribution in claimant and normative samples. (*G*) Communication and cognition scale distribution in claimant and normative samples.

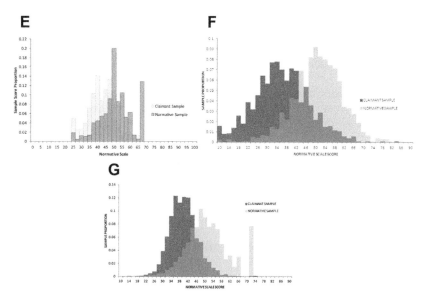

Fig. 3. (continued).

the mental health domains of the WB-FAB, the goal was to expand the scope of work disability assessment by creating a measure of functional, activity-based aspects relevant to a person's potential ability to work. This research integrates a more functional approach into the paradigm of work disability assessment, focusing on activities or tasks that relate to a person's potential ability to participate in the workplace compared with more traditional definitions of disability.

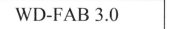

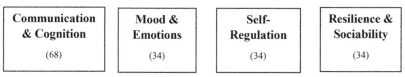

Fig. 4. WD-FAB_{3.0} domain and items.

Second, instruments like the WD-FAB, developed using IRT methodology, are "dynamic" in that the WD-FAB's use of IRT/CAT methods allow for updating and improvement over time. Updated forms of the WD-FAB can be created from the existing item bank while maintaining the underlying measurement metric. This unique feature of IRT methods allows for future WD-FAB versions to be comparable with earlier versions. Best practice in work disability assessment is constantly changing, so having an assessment instrument that can be updated to reflect current scientific and conceptual views on work-related disability has the potential to be a valuable resource for

Identifier: MOCKUP1   Date: 1/15/18

Gender: Female   Age: 30

Primary Allegation: Chronic Low Back Pain

Physical Function Profile	Score Estimate	Score Precision
Basic Mobility: Involves getting into and out of positions, staying in positions for periods of time, and walking and moving around from one place to another.	25	±4
Upper Body Function: Involves using arms and body to push, pull, and carry objects and move them from one place to another.	48	±4
Fine Motor Function: Involves the coordinated actions of handling objects, picking up, manipulating, and releasing them using one's hand, fingers, and thumb.	52	±4
Public Transportation: Involves using buses, trains, or subways to get from one place to another; this includes using timetables, wayfinding, and getting in and out of train cars or buses.	45	±4
Driving: Planning and carrying out the tasks involved in driving a motor vehicle, such as entering/exiting, navigating roadways, and parking.	60	±4

Mental Health Function Domains	Score Estimate	Score Precision
Mood & Emotions represents a range of aspects of a person's internal emotional state that can affect a person's ability to work, including degree of emotional stability, depressive feelings, and anxiety.	30	±4
Resilience & Sociability includes a range of capabilities related to handling stress, accomplishing goals, and learning from mistakes. Resilience is the process of adapting well in the face of adversity, trauma, tragedy, threats, or significant sources of stress — such as family and relationship problems, serious health problems or workplace and financial stressors.	50	±4
Self-Regulation characterizes attributes of function, such as controlling temper, respecting others, following rules, social abilities, interacting with people in a contextually appropriate manner, and responding to the feelings of others.	55	±4
Cognition & Communication includes aspects of function, such as organizational skills, attention, following instructions, oral and written communication, applying knowledge that is learned, thinking, solving problems, and making decisions.	60	±4

Fig. 5. WD-FAB functional profile.

a wide array of stakeholders who are interested in systematically and efficiently assessing work-related physical and mental health functioning. The efficiencies gained by the CAT administration while preserving the breadth of content coverage allow for potential policy relevant and clinical applications of the WD-FAB.

Practically, the WD-FAB can be used to generate functional profiles for an individual along several key dimensions of physical and mental health function that are important for work. A simple example can illustrate how the WD-FAB can be used to create individual functional profiles. **Fig. 5** illustrates the WD-FAB functional profile for a 30-year-old woman with chronic back pain who has applied for work disability benefits. The WD-FAB displays this woman's physical function profile in 4 domains: basic mobility, upper-body function, fine-motor function, and community mobility (public transportation and driving), and her mental health function in 4 domains: mood and emotions, resilience and sociability, self-regulation and communication, and cognition. Each WD-FAB score is an estimate of a person's function in relation to an average standard score of 50 derived from the working-age adult population in the United States and a standard deviation around the person's score, where 1 standard deviation is ±10 points. The profile in **Fig. 5** indicates this woman has severe limitations in basic mobility function with a score of 25, 2.5 standard deviations below the average score for a working-age population. She also has a score of 30 in mood and emotions, also well below the population mean. Her functional profile is within the average range for the other functional domains.

As this example illustrates, the WD-FAB scales can be used to create multidimensional functional profiles of persons applying for work disability benefits and can be compared with scores for a general US working-age adult sample. Such profiles could be used to inform work disability adjudication decisions, treatment planning for rehabilitation, and subsequent return to work decisions, as well as identifying work environments where work requirements match the functional profile of the individual.

From initial work disability screening to reevaluation of disability status, there is clear potential for the WD-FAB to play an important role in improving disability assessment within the context of work disability programs as well as within other clinical and vocational rehabilitation settings. The WD-FAB is a tool that has the ability to provide data to support and improve decision making around work disability assessment. In addition, the WD-FAB could be informative for guiding clinical care targeting return to work interventions as well as assist vocational rehabilitation counselors to identify areas of strengths and weaknesses in their goal of matching underlying functional ability with potential job demands of the work environment.

REFERENCES

1. IOM. The future of disability in America. In: Fields M, Jette AM, editors. Washington, DC: The National Academies Press; 2007.
2. Institute on Disability. 2015 annual disability statistics compendium. Durham (NH): University of New Hampshire; 2016.
3. Brandt DE, Houtenville AJ, Huynh M, et al. Connecting contemporary paradigms to social security administration's disability evaluation process. J Disabil Policy Stud 2011;20:1–13.
4. Masala C, Petretto DR. From disablement to enablement: conceptual models of disability in the 20th century. Disabil Rehabil 2008;30:1233–44.
5. World Health Organization. International classification of functioning, disability and health. Geneva (Switzerland): World Health Organization; 2001.

6. Escorpizo R, Gmunder HP, Stucki G. Introduction to special section: advancing the field of vocational rehabilitation with the international classification of functioning, disability and health (ICF). J Occup Rehabil 2011;21(2):121–5.

7. Anthony WA, Rogers ES, Cohen M, et al. Relationships between psychiatric symptomatology, work skills, and future vocational performance. Psychiatr Serv 1995;46:353–84.

8. MacDonald-Wilson KL, Rogers ES, Anthony WA. Unique issues in assessing work function among individuals with psychiatric disabilities. J Occup Rehabil 2001; 11(3):217–32.

9. Wideman TH, Sullivan MJ. Differential predictors of the long-term levels of pain intensity, work disability, healthcare use, and medication use in a sample of workers' compensation claimants. Pain 2011;152:376–83.

10. D'Amato A, Zijlstra F. Toward a climate for work resumption: the nonmedical determinants of return to work. J Occup Environ Med 2010;52:67–80.

11. Marfeo EE, Haley SM, Jette AM, et al. A conceptual foundation for measures of physical function and behavioral health function for Social Security work disability evaluation. Arch Phys Med Rehabil 2013;94:1645–52.e2.

12. McDonough CM, Jette AM, Ni P, et al. Development of a self-report physical function instrument for disability assessment: item pool construction and factor analysis. Arch Phys Med Rehabil 2013;94(9):1653–60.

13. Ni PS, McDonough CM, Jette AM, et al. Development of a computer-adaptive physical function instrument for Social Security Administration disability determination. Arch Phys Med Rehabil 2013;94:1661–9.

14. Marfeo EE, Ni P, Haley SM, et al. Development of an instrument to measure behavioral health function for work disability: item pool construction and factor analysis. Arch Phys Med Rehabil 2013;94(9):1670–80.

15. Marfeo EE, Ni P, Haley SM, et al. Scale refinement and initial evaluation of a behavioral health function measurement tool for work disability evaluation. Arch Phys Med Rehabil 2013;94(9):1679–86.

16. Green BF, Bock RD, Humphreys LG, et al. Technical guidelines for assessing computerized adaptive tests. J Educ Meas 1984;21:347–60.

17. Meterko M, Marfeo EE, McDonough CM, et al. Work disability functional assessment battery: feasibility and psychometric properties. Arch Phys Med Rehabil 2015;96(6):1028–35.

18. Marino ME, Meterko M, Marfeo EE, et al. Work related measures of physical and behavioral health function: test-retest reliability. Disabil Health J 2015;8(4):652–7.

19. Haley S, Ni P, Jette A, et al. Replenishing a computerized adaptive test of patient-reported daily activity functioning. Qual Life Res 2009;18(4):461–71.

20. McDonough CM, Ni P, Peterik K, et al. Improving measures of work-related physical functioning. Qual Life Res 2017;26(3):789–98.

21. Marfeo EE, Ni P, McDonough C, et al. Improving assessment of work related mental health function using the work disability functional assessment battery (WD-FAB). J Occup Rehabil 2018;28(1):190–9.

Measuring Burden of Care After Catastrophic Illness or Injury

Paulette M. Niewczyk, MPH, PhD[a,b,]*

KEYWORDS

- Burden of care • FIM® • LIFEware System • Northwick Park Dependency Scale
- Outcomes measurement

KEY POINTS

- Burden of care (BoC) is the amount of time a patient requires direct assistance from another person each day to meet basic needs in the home; BoC it is based on a patient's functional level, obtained using the Functional Independence Measure instrument.
- BoC is used for patient assessment, for hospital discharge planning, and to communicate care needs with patients and families.
- The Northwick Park Dependency Scale can be used to quantify a patient's need for nursing care and daily support during a stay in an inpatient facility or home-based care needs for persons receiving home health care or outpatient care in community-based settings.
- The LIFEware System can be used to monitor function and BoC in the outpatient setting.

THE NEED TO MEASURE OUTCOMES

For more than 2 decades, a nationwide effort has been directed to assess and improve the quality of health care in the United States. The Institute of Medicine (IOM) instigated this effort in 1996 as a result of research to investigate access to care, delivery of services, and quality of health care received. As a result of the research, the IOM published a report that stated a need for creating, implementing, and reporting measures to determine how well health care is delivered.[1] The report stated that the US

Disclosures: P. Niewczyk is employed by Uniform Data System for Medical Rehabilitation. No commercial or financial conflicts of interest associated with this work; the article was written without funding or any financial remuneration.
FIM® and LIFEware^SM are registered to Uniform Data System for Medical Rehabilitation, a division of UB Foundations Activities, Inc.
[a] Uniform Data System for Medical Rehabilitation, University at Buffalo, 270 Northpointe Parkway, Suite 300, Amherst, NY 14228, USA; [b] Department of Health Promotion, Daemen College, Amherst, NY, USA
* Uniform Data System for Medical Rehabilitation, 270 Northpointe Parkway, Suite 300, Amherst, NY 14228.
E-mail address: pniewczyk@udsmr.org

Phys Med Rehabil Clin N Am 30 (2019) 573–580
https://doi.org/10.1016/j.pmr.2019.03.005
1047-9651/19/© 2019 Elsevier Inc. All rights reserved.

health care system rewards overuse of services and the frequent use of high-cost complex procedures and does not account for the wide variations in quality across providers.[1] The report concluded that care reforms are needed and set a long-term goal for the health care system to provide care that is safe, effective, patient-centered, timely, efficient, and equitable.[2]

MEASURING PATIENT PHYSICAL AND COGNITIVE FUNCTIONING: THE FUNCTIONAL INDEPENDENCE MEASUREINSTRUMENT

Long before the IOM report was published, program evaluation was a routine, ongoing function within a large proportion of the inpatient rehabilitation field. Many clinicians in inpatient rehabilitation facilities (IRFs) nationwide already were routinely examining outcomes of care, quality of care, and utilization of services at both the patient and facility levels using objective measures, such as the Functional Independence Measure (FIM®) instrument. Effectiveness, efficiency, timeliness, resource use, and safety are an integral part of the FIM® instrument, which was developed by the Uniform Data System for Medical Rehabilitation (UDSMR) in 1987 for use in measuring, tracking, and reporting patient and facility rehabilitation outcomes to guide and improve quality of care. Since 2002, the FIM® has been used for program management as well as payment by rehabilitation clinicians on every Medicare-insured patient admitted and discharged from an IRF because the measure is embedded in the Centers for Medicare and Medicaid Services IRF Patient Assessment Instrument (PAI). Additionally, a majority of IRF clinicians routinely use the FIM® instrument to assess function and outcomes in non-Medicare patients.

The IRF-PAI was implemented in 2002 and currently serves as the basis for Medicare reimbursement under the inpatient rehabilitation prospective payment system. Through the UDSMR, the IRF-PAI also serves a program evaluation function in that it allows for ongoing monitoring of patient outcomes and comparison of outcomes across all inpatient medical rehabilitation facilities in the United States.

A component of the IRF-PAI, the FIM® instrument, is an additive scale comprising 13 physical/motor function items and 5 cognitive function items, each rated on a 7-level, ordinal scale measuring degree of dependence and need for helper assistance. The IRF-PAI supplements the items of the FIM® instrument with diagnostic information, personal support information, and certain quality indicators included as federal mandates.

The FIM® instrument has a high overall internal consistency, can capture significant functional gains during rehabilitation, has high discriminative capabilities for rehabilitation patients, and is a good indicator of patient burden of care (BoC).[3,4] FIM® ratings differ depending on the medical conditions of patients[3]; additionally, the instrument discriminates among patients on the basis of age, comorbidity, and discharge destination.[4] Validation research confirmed the FIM® accurately predicted patient care needs and length of acute rehabilitation stay, and the instrument can be used to predict inpatient utilization and approximate length of stay in inpatient rehabilitation.[4]

The FIM® instrument is a standardized, fixed-item assessment instrument, developed based on classical test theory (CTT). CTT uses standardized psychometric procedures to develop a fixed set of questions (or items) to measure a given, unidimensional construct (such as function) selected on the basis of appropriateness for a targeted population (such as patients admitted to an IRF) but unrelated to any specific impairment, condition, trait, or disease (applicable for a wide range of functional impairments/conditions).

It has been argued that CTT-based assessments should be replaced by a test administration method, known as computer adaptive testing (CAT).[5] CAT-based assessment instruments are constructed using a measurement theory, known as item response theory, the methods of which examine the associations between individuals' responses to a series of items designed to measure a specific outcome domain (eg, functional status).[6] An algorithm is used to select test items tailored to an individual patient, shortens or lengthens the test to achieve the desired precision of measurement, scores every patient on the same underlying outcome continuum so that results can be compared across the continuum of that outcome, and displays the results instantly for immediate interpretation and use.[5]

CAT-based assessments have been widely used in educational testing as with the Graduate Record Examination (GRE) and for diagnostic needs assessment but have less applicability for use in managing patient care.[7] CAT-based assessments, however, do not allow for direct comparability between participants, or even within the same participant tested.[6] Because items administered through CAT are derived from a large item bank, 2 participants may be administered items with similar levels of difficulty but it may not be the exact question administered to each person; this has an impact on data standardization.[6] Additionally, because therapists may be targeting certain functional impairments (such as ambulation, dressing self, gait, and balance) in a patient, it is imperative to be able to assess the specific functional domain at multiple times during a patient's IRF stay to ensure progress and functional gain. If the same item is not addressed over time, this provides a large challenge to the clinician in monitoring patient progress and outcomes of care. Standard fixed tests provide the best precision for average-level ability and less precision for extreme test scores, or outliers.[8] In other words, when it is anticipated that there is a wide range of abilities, from the extreme low to the extreme high, CAT-based testing is preferred to standard fixed tests. In the IRF, typical patients have some functional impairment but must be strong enough to participate in intensive therapy defined as 3 hours per day of interdisciplinary therapy at least 5 days per week. Patients who are too frail, debilitated, or very low functioning (extreme low functioning) are not typically candidates for admission to an IRF and certainly those who are very high functioning and have mild functional deficits (eg. post–sport-related injury or post–elective outpatient surgery) do not warrant admission to inpatient care (extreme high functioning); therefore, CAT-based testing is not an ideal method for measuring functional outcomes of patients treated in inpatient rehabilitation.

MEASURING PATIENT BURDEN OF CARE

The main goals of rehabilitation are to restore functional ability (when possible) and to minimize the extent of functional impairment, limitations, and disability; to improve patient quality of life; and to discharge patients back to home or a community-based setting. Improvements in a patient's ability to self-care and perform activities of daily living independently or with the least amount of assistance needed from a caregiver are essential to be able to discharge patients to their home or the home of a family member. Improving a patient's function reduces the BoC on a patient's caregivers, which increases the likelihood of the patient's return to home or community and reduces the risk of an acute readmission and/or need for extended inpatient long-term care.

UDSMR developed a common metric, called BoC, which is the estimated amount of time, in hours, that an individual needs 1-on-1 assistance from another person (family member, health care provider, or spouse) to perform routine activities of daily living (grooming, dressing, ambulation, walking/moving, and social interaction) and meet basic self-care needs (eating, toileting, bathing, expressing/communicating needs, and problem solving) in a home-based setting each day. The BoC is based on an individual's physical and cognitive functional levels, which are obtained from an assessment using the FIM® instrument. Based on the individual's total 18-item FIM® score, the range of FIM® ratings correspond to an approximate total number of hours an individual will need 1-on-1 assistance daily from a caregiver. BoC can be used to aid in hospital triage decisions for acute care and post–acute care discharge planning and as a tool for communicating with patients and their families regarding the individual's care needs and estimated time each day of 1-on-1 caregiving assistance that would be required in the home or community-based setting. **Table 1** displays the range of total FIM® scores based on the 18-item FIM® assessment and the corresponding estimated time in hours for each level of functioning.

The FIM® instrument has been validated as a measure of BoC by several studies that were conducted correlating individuals FIM® scores with the amount of time actually spent (using a stopwatch each time assistance was provided and recording time spent in minutes) by caregivers in the community providing direct assistance to the individual. A strong, significant correlation between total FIM® score and amount of time needed for assistance from a caregiver was found in multiple prospective studies.[9–13] BoC is applicable for use in the acute care hospital and for all inpatient post–acute care settings.[14] Additionally, the FIM® instrument can be used for individuals with physical and/or cognitive impairment requiring outpatient or home-based care to determine the BOC and extent of services that will be needed (eg, licensed practical nurse [LPN]/registered nurse [RN]/physical therapist/occupational therapist/additional therapeutic services) for the individual to be safely cared for at home or in a community-based residential setting.

MEASURING INPATIENT BURDEN OF CARE: THE NORTHWICK PARK DEPENDENCY SCALE

Inpatient BoC is the projected resources that will be needed to care for a patient during an inpatient stay (eg, number of nursing hours required to provide daily care, need for specialized providers, and nursing level/intensity needed). The Northwick Park Dependency Scale (NPDS) was developed in Great Britain for use in nursing and rehabilitation settings to quantify inpatient BoC, defined as an individual's need for nursing care and daily support.[15] The assessment tool includes activities of daily living, safety

Table 1	
Burden of care: amount of assistance needed from a caregiver based on level of functioning	
Functional Independence Measure Score: Range of Scores	**Hours of Direct Caregiver Assistance Needed per Day**
18–30	≥8
31–53	6–7
54–71	4–5
72–89	2–3
90–107	1–2
108–119	<1
120–126	0[a]

[a] Not an absolute zero; the patient may require assistance from a caregiver but it is minimal in time (a couple of times a week or only a few minutes each day).

awareness, behavioral management, and communication. The NPDS score quantifies an individual's nursing care needs in post–acute care and home/community-based settings by yielding an estimate of care hours and approximate cost of care required. The NPDS provides information about the individual's particular nursing needs in terms of number of caregivers required per day, need for specialized nurses, and need for cognitive and behavioral nursing management. The tool is applicable for use on all impairment types, whereby it is intended to be used with any patient requiring inpatient or home-based nursing care.

The NPDS is an ordinal measure, with scores ranging from 0 to 100 and divided into 2 sections: a Basic Care Needs section (ranging from 0 to 65), which includes 16 items associated with activities of daily living, and a Special Nursing Needs section (ranging from 0 to 35), which includes 7 dichotomous items related to need for specially trained nursing care. The NPDS total score is interpreted based on 4 levels of dependency: 0 to 9 = low dependency, 10 to 24 = medium dependency, 25 to 40 = high dependency, and greater than 40 = very high dependency.

The NPDS has been studied in rehabilitation settings alongside other measures of dependency, including the FIM® instrument, and was found to correlate well with the other functional dependency tools.[16] The NPDS differs from the FIM® instrument and other functional instruments in that the NPDS is intended to assess BoC from a nursing perspective, whereby the individual's level of functioning is a component but not the primary purpose of the assessment, unlike the FIM® instrument, which is centered on capturing an individual's physical and cognitive function and need for assistance from a caregiver. The NPDS has been found to have good internal consistency, to discriminate among persons with different dependency levels, and to be responsive to change, particularly in the higher dependency/more severe patient population.[17]

MEASURING FUNCTION IN OUTPATIENT SETTINGS: THE LIFEware SYSTEM

At the outpatient level, determining an individual's care plan and setting goals typically start with an assessment of the individual's functional status and medical needs, which can be assessed using the LIFEware System. Additionally, the LIFEware System can be used to assess an individual's change in function (improvement/worsening) over the course of outpatient treatment, to evaluate therapy effectiveness, and to monitor the need for continuing care. The LIFEware System contains more than 130 different functional outcome assessment instruments to comprehensively evaluate physical function, cognitive function, mood, pain, social interaction, activity participation, quality of life, and satisfaction with treatment of patients with all types of impairments/conditions requiring outpatient rehabilitation.[18] There are patient-reported measures and clinician-assessed instruments within the LIFEware System, which are used by the treating clinician to track the functional status of patients over the course of care. The clinician selects the instruments and measures that best meet the particular needs of a given patient, so if 1 patient receives frequent, short-term (eg, 3 times per week for 12 weeks) outpatient physical therapy and occupational therapy poststroke, measures, such as body movement and control, locomotion, and activities of daily living, may be selected, whereas another patient within the same outpatient therapy center may receive extended, long-term (1 time per week, ongoing) physical therapy for symptoms associated with multiple sclerosis, measures, such as multiple sclerosis physical functioning, Expanded Disability Status Scale,[19] and visual analog scale,[20] may be selected to monitor patient outcomes and functional improvement over the duration of treatment.

The measures contained within the LIFEware System have been validated using Rasch analysis, a statistical method used to assess the psychometric properties of an assessment tool.[21] Rasch analysis was used to recalibrate all measures within the LIFEware System so measures using ordinal ratings are converted to interval-like properties and each measure is on the same range of scores, from 0 to 100, where a higher score is better functioning.[22] By recalibrating each measure, different instruments can be compared in terms of outcomes and functional improvement, even if the instruments contain a different number of questions or have different rating scale for items (Likert vs binary). Additionally, benchmarks are established for each measure based on individual assessment data from more than 300,000 outpatients followed longitudinally whereby an expected level of functioning is provided for each measure based on the mathematical average of all patients with the same medical condition requiring care. In essence, this serves as a norm-based reference value so the clinician can determine the extent of functional impairment for a particular patient based on that patient's actual scores compared with the expected score (the mathematical average score for all patients with the same medical condition); this reference value also can help in patient goal setting at the start of care and to aid in clinical evaluation to establish new therapy goals over the course of care based on patient change in functioning from one point in time to the next.[23]

The LIFEware System has been found reliable and valid for outpatient use and is applicable to many different impairments and conditions, including but not limited to, stroke,[12] multiple sclerosis,[11] traumatic brain injury,[24] pain management,[25] coronary disease,[26] and musculoskeletal problems.[27,28]

MOVING FORWARD: MEASURING PATIENT OUTCOMES AMID MANY DIFFERENT MEASURES

Measuring and monitoring outcomes of all care result in reduced health care expenditures, more streamlined patient care, and improved quality of life for patients and their families. As previously discussed, there are many different instruments that can be used to measure patient function, therapeutic needs, amount of caregiver assistance needed for daily living tasks, and outcomes of care/changes in function. The aforementioned instruments are just a few that have been heavily researched and widely used for decades; there are many more instruments available for use. As previously established, it is important to measure outcomes of care but it is equally important to select the best instrument to assess and capture the specific outcome of interest, in the setting and/or for the patient population/type that the instrument was designed to assess. Unfortunately, a best, all-encompassing, highly reliable, and valid instrument to measure patient outcomes of care does not exist, at least not at the present time. Many instruments, with a range in reliability and validity, are available, and some of these tools, which seem equal in terms of reliability and validity, are better at capturing some outcomes than others, are more precise in some settings than others, or are able to detect changes in some patient populations but not within a general population. In essence, the best instrument truly depends on the overarching purpose or intention for use. For instance, if trying to determine actual nursing care needs, such as level/type of care (LPN vs RN vs Certified Rehabilitation Registered Nurse [CRRN]) and amount duration of care required in terms of hours per day of nursing care, then the NPDS would be better than the Barthel index[29] or the FIM®. If the purpose is to determine if an individual has any functional impairment (qualifying for services or need for care), the Barthel index and the FIM® would be best suited because these instruments offer a more comprehensive assessment of an individual's level of functioning. If the purpose is to assess an individual's change in function (improvement/worsening, therapy effectiveness, or need for continuing care) over time (days, weeks, or more), the FIM® would be better than the NPDS and the Barthel index, because the FIM® rating is more sensitive to detect change in function, whereby the FIM® includes 7 levels in the rating scale opposed to the Barthel index, which includes only 3 rating levels, and the NPDS, in which only 2 levels (dichotomous) are used with many of the items.

SUMMARY

A great deal of variability has been found among providers, hospitals, IRFs, skilled nursing homes, and other long-term care settings based on effectiveness, efficiency, patient outcomes, and quality of care. Measuring and monitoring outcomes of all care will result in reduced health care expenditures, more streamlined patient care, and improved quality of life for patients and their families, closer to achieving the IOM goal of getting the right patient to the right setting at the right time. Rehabilitation patients are the ultimate beneficiaries of improvements in standards of care as they increasingly strive for outcomes that allow them to live independently with the least amount of assistance from a caregiver in noninstitutional settings without placing a strain on family members or friends.

REFERENCES

1. Institute of Medicine. Priority areas for national action: transforming health care quality. Washington, DC: The National Academies Press; 2003. https://doi.org/10.17226/10593.
2. English WJ. Rewarding provider performance: aligning incentives in Medicare. Ann Intern Med 2008;148:636.
3. Heinemann AW, Linacre JM, Wright BD, et al. Relationships between impairment and physical disability as measured by the Functional Independence Measure. Arch Phys Med Rehabil 1993;74(6):566–73.
4. Stineman MG, Shea JD, Jette A, et al. The functional independence measure: tests of scaling assumptions, structure, and reliability across 20 diverse impairment categories. Arch Phys Med Rehabil 1996;77(11):1101–8.
5. Jette A, Haley SM, Ni P. Comparison of functional status tools used in post-acute care. Health Care Financ Rev 2003;24(3):13–24.
6. Weiss D, Kingsbury G. Application of computerized adaptive testing to educational problems. J Edu Meas 1984;21(4):361–75.
7. Ware JE, Bjorner JB, Kosinski M. Practical implications of item response theory and computerized adaptive testing: a brief summary of ongoing studies of widely used Headache Impact Scales. Med Care 2000;39(S9):473–83.
8. Thissen D, Mislevy RJ. Testing algorithms. In: Wainer H, editor. Computerized adaptive testing: a primer. Mahwah (NJ): Lawrence Erlbaum Associates; 2000. p. 101–33.
9. Corrigan JD, Smith-Knapp K, Granger CV. Validity of the functional independence measure for persons with traumatic brain injury. Arch Phys Med Rehabil 1997; 78(8):828–34.
10. Disler PB, Roy CW, Smith BP. Predicting hours of care needed. Arch Phys Med Rehabil 1993;74(2):139–43.
11. Granger CV, Cotter AC, Hamilton BB, et al. Functional assessment scales: a study of persons with multiple sclerosis. Arch Phys Med Rehabil 1990;71(11):870–5.

12. Granger CV, Cotter AC, Hamilton BB, et al. Functional assessment scales: a study of persons after stroke. Arch Phys Med Rehabil 1993;74(2):133–8.
13. Hamilton BB, Deutsch A, Russell C, et al. Relation of disability costs to function: spinal cord injury. Arch Phys Med Rehabil 1999;80(4):385–91.
14. Stillman G, Granger CV, Niewczyk P. Projecting function of stroke patients in rehabilitation using the AlphaFIM instrument in acute care. PM R 2009;1(3):234–9.
15. Turner-Stokes L, Tonge P, Nyein K, et al. The Northwick Park Dependency Score (NPDS): a measure of nursing dependency in rehabilitation. Clin Rehabil 1998; 12(4):304–18.
16. Turner-Stokes L, Williams H, Rose H, et al. Deriving a Barthel Index from the Northwick Park Dependency Scale and the Functional Independence measure – are they equivalent? Clin Rehabil 2010;24(12):1121–6.
17. Siegert RJ, Turner-Stokes L. Psychometric evaluation of the Northwick Park Dependency Scale. J Rehabil Med 2010;42(10):936–43.
18. Granger CV, Linn RT. Biologic patterns of disability. J Outcome Meas 2000;4(2): 595–615.
19. Kurtzke JF. Rating neurologic impairment in multiple sclerosis: an Expanded Disability Status Scale (EDSS). Neurology 1983;33(11):1444–52.
20. Wewers ME, Lowe NK. A critical review of visual analog scales in the measurement of clinical phenomena. Res Nurs Health 1990;13(4):227–36.
21. Baker JG, Granger CV, Fiedler RC. A brief outpatient functional assessment measure: validity using Rasch measures. Am J Phys Med Rehabil 1997;7:8–13.
22. Granger CV, Carlin M. The LIFEware system and rasch analysis: evaluating functional status of multiple sclerosis patients. In: Bezruczko N, editor. Rasch measurement in health sciences. Maple Grove (MN): JAM Press; 2005. p. 260–76.
23. Baker JG, Fiedler RC, Ottenbacher KJ, et al. Predicting follow-up functional outcomes in outpatient rehabilitation. Am J Phys Med Rehabil 1998;77(3):202–12.
24. Granger CV, Divan N, Fiedler RC. Functional assessment scales: a study of persons after traumatic brain injury. Am J Phys Med Rehabil 1995;74(2):107–13.
25. Tesio L, Granger CV, Fiedler RC. A unidimentional pain/disability measure for low back pain syndromes. Pain 1997;69:269–78.
26. Mithal M, Mann WC, Granger CV. The role of coronary heart disease (CHD) in functional limitation in community dwelling elders. Phys Occup Ther Geriatr 2001;19(3):35–47.
27. Linn RT, Granger CV, Disler PB, et al. Applications of functional assessment to musculoskeletal disability evaluation. Phys Med Rehabil Clin N Am 2001;12(3): 529–41.
28. Granger CV, Lackner JM, Kulas M, et al. Outpatients with low back pain: an analysis of the rate per day of pain improvement that may be expected and factors affecting improvement. Am J Phys Med Rehabil 2003;82:253–60.
29. Mahoney F, Barthel D. Functional evaluation: the barthel index. Md Med J 1965; 14:61–5.

Burden of Treatment Compliance as an Impairment Rating Metric

Stephen L. Demeter, MD, MPH

KEYWORDS

- BOTC • Burden of treatment compliance • Activities of daily living (ADLs)
- Surrogate • Static • Functional

KEY POINTS

- All editions of the American Medical Association (AMA) guides traditionally rate impairment based on static deviations from population or personal norms in addition to rating based on interferences in activities of daily living (ADLs).
- The burden of treatment compliance (BOTC) method of impairment rating was developed as a stand-alone model to help overcome difficulties when rating internal medicine conditions, when normative metrics may be lacking and impacts on ADLs are not readily determined.
- With the changes in the sixth edition of the AMA guides, the BOTC model has been adapted to provide alternative operational metrics for functional losses associated with these conditions.

HISTORICAL DEVELOPMENT

The most common problems rated using the American Medical Association (AMA) guides are orthopedic injuries. Despite the frequency, all editions of the guides have provided ratings for not just orthopedic injuries but also for medical injuries/illnesses, problems affecting the vision and hearing, psychiatric conditions, and (starting with the guide's fourth edition[1]) pain. When rating an orthopedic injury, the injury can be rated using the anatomic deviation (a static condition) or the associated interferences with activities of daily living (ADLs) (a functional or dynamic condition).

The most difficult conditions to assess by this conventional rating approach are pain and mental-behavioral impairments. Pain (defined as the perception of nociception) is by nature a purely subjective issue and, therefore, is not readily amenable to objective measurement–based testing. Psychiatric issues are just starting to be amenable to objective measurement testing. Examples include emotional and memory changes

---

Disclosure: The author has nothing to disclose.
2925 Josephine Drive, Henderson, NV 89044, USA
E-mail address: stevedemeter96825@gmail.com

Phys Med Rehabil Clin N Am 30 (2019) 581–587
https://doi.org/10.1016/j.pmr.2019.03.006
1047-9651/19/© 2019 Elsevier Inc. All rights reserved.

that can be seen as abnormalities on an MRI scan. However, these have yet to evolve into tests that are sufficiently reliable to be used for diagnosis, treatment, and prognosis and, hence, an impairment rating.

Impairments of the special senses (eg, hearing and vision) have sufficient objective testing to allow ratings for functional impairments, with a few notable exceptions. For example, tinnitus cannot be objectively verified and the rating is entirely based on subjective criteria.

Internal medicine impairment ratings may involve the following organ systems: cardiovascular, pulmonary, gastrointestinal (including hernias), genitourinary, dermatologic, hematopoietic, endocrinologic, and neurologic. For such organ systems, static parameters may be easily defined and applied. For example, a person can have an abnormal electrocardiogram or echocardiogram whereby left ventricular hypertrophy might be identified. However, how does this relate to a cardiovascular functional impairment? A pulmonary function test is a static test; it does not test exercise capacity. Exercise capacity is tested using a cardiopulmonary exercise stress test that relates, directly, to functional impairment. This impairment translates into interferences in the ADLs. For example, if a person has a forced expiratory volume in 1 second of 29% of predicted, there is a significant deviation from normalcy. This measure is a static test. It suggests, but does not prove, significant functional impairment. An exercise stress test can show the functional or dynamic impairment. Multiple references could be provided showing tables that describe exercise capabilities based on the results of the exercise stress test.[2–5]

Not all organ systems are amenable to the assessment of functional capability. If a person has nerve conduction velocity and electromyogram findings showing moderate to severe carpal tunnel syndrome, how does this correlate with interferences in that person's ADLs? If a person has peptic ulcer disease and has continued symptoms at maximal medical improvement, how does this correlate with functional impairment? If a person has osteoporosis, how much functional impairment is created by this condition?

Questions such as these have prompted the adoption of an alternative approach for rating internal medicine issues according to the AMA guides. How do clinicians begin to rate issues such as congestive heart failure, diabetes, irritable bowel syndrome, and hypertension? In most cases, static tests are all that is available and these are being supplemented by subjective reporting, which can have validity, reliability, and other concerns. Is there a better way, or at least an alternative way, of assessing impairment for internal medicine conditions?

One principle frequently found in the treatment of internal medicine conditions is the concept of the use of multiple medications. The number of medications used is often a reflection of the severity of the condition. For example, if a person has very mild hypertension, a single antihypertensive medication may be all that is necessary to control the condition. If the hypertension is of greater intensity (moderate or severe), or difficult to treat, then multiple medications may be necessary. These medications may be taken once a day or more frequently.

Medications may create side effects and/or potential disturbances that need to be corrected. There may be little functional impairment associated with treatment of mild hypertension managed with an angiotensin-converting enzyme (ACE) inhibitor medication once a day. In contrast, patients with very severe hypertension may take a calcium channel blocker 3 times a day, an ACE inhibitor twice a day, and 2 different diuretics with supplemental potassium. There may be dietary restrictions as well. It would seem that the number of medications, the frequency of medication usage, the treatment of potential side effects of those medications, and other factors such as the dietary restrictions can provide the basis for a useful metric to determine and grade the severity of a given medical condition.

The burden of treatment compliance (BOTC) rating metric was developed to address these issues. This metric allowed an assessment of impairment rating for medical conditions based on medication usage, frequency, and side effects. It further allowed the assessment of impairment based on interferences in ADLs caused by either the ratable condition, the treatment of the ratable condition, or other interferences caused by the ratable condition (such as dietary changes). In addition, it allowed for the possibility of problems created by a treatment or procedure (for example, radiation therapy or an exploratory laparotomy) that might be too mild to otherwise rate (for example, cramps 3 or 4 times a week caused by adhesions from a laparotomy). One of the principal components of the BOTC was the qualitative and quantitative use of medications as a surrogate for the severity of the condition. Another component was allowing the interferences in the ADLs to be a driving force for determining the impairment.

Consider Mr Alpha who is 29 years old and has type I diabetes. As result of his condition, he takes insulin and oral medications. His current regimen consists of checking his blood sugar 4 times a day, taking an oral hypoglycemic medication once a day, taking a second oral hypoglycemic medication twice a day, injecting a long-acting insulin preparation once a day, and supplementing his insulin injections with a short-acting preparation 3 times a day approximately 30 minutes before each meal. As a result of his diabetic condition, this man has an impairment. He has both a static impairment (a deviation from population norms; ie, the diabetes) and a functional impairment (the treatments necessitated by his medical condition that cause interferences in his ADLs).

The BOTC addresses functional interferences, namely interferences in an individual's ADLs created by the impairing condition. It does not address static issues even though, in the example given earlier, there is a static condition, namely diabetes mellitus. The static condition is not ratable, per se, because it relies on the treatment and the interferences in a person's ADLs created by the treatments, the modalities of the treatments, the dietary alterations, and other issues, which is seen in the amount of time, energy, and inconvenience Mr Alpha must spend each day in caring for his diabetic condition.

BOTC reflects how much interference in a person's ADLs are created by directly taking care of the injury or illness when at maximal medical improvement. If it is significant, then those interferences create a burden on the individual.

For example, Ms Beta has hypertension and takes a single medication once a day. Is there any significant interference in her ADLs from taking a pill once a day? The answer is most likely not. Her husband, who also has hypertension, takes multiple medications and adheres to a low-salt, low-cholesterol, and low-caloric-intake diet. Are there significant interferences in his ADLs? The answer is most likely yes.

When examining the issue of BOTC, a variety of criteria are used to reflect interferences with ADLs. These criteria are found in Appendix B of the sixth edition[6(pp607,608)] and are extrapolated into the following criteria:

1. The number of medications taken to control the subject injury/illness when at maximal medical improvement
2. The frequency and timing of a medication administration; these are seen below in order from easiest to hardest:
   a. At any time
   b. Once a day

    c. Twice a day

    d. Three times a day

    e. Four times a day

    f. Before or after an event, such as a meal

3. Ease of a medication administration; these are seen below in order from easiest to hardest:

    a. Oral administration

    b. Dermal administration; for example, creams and salves (unless extensive, in which case it would be lower on this list)

    c. Intranasal administration

    d. Ocular administration

    e. Inhaled administration

    f. Rectal administration

    g. Injections; from easiest to hardest:

        i. Subcutaneous

        ii. Intradermal

        iii. Intramuscular

        iv. Intravenous

        v. Intracavitary

        vi. Intrathecal

4. Dietary modifications

5. Side effects and complications routinely experienced as a result of medications and/or treatments (for example, the need to urinate 10–12 times per day because of a diuretic)

6. Frequency of routinely performed procedures; for example, emptying urine or fecal collective devices, the use of compressive hose, the care of peripherally inserted cutaneous catheter lines

In addition, other issues are discussed, including:

1. If a combination medication is used, then the condition is assessed by the total number of medications. For example, if an antihypertensive medication is used that is combined with a diuretic, then the medication is counted twice because side effects potentially accrue from each medication.

2. If the BOTC is applied, then the medication and/or treatment must pertain to the subject injury or illness. However, if the medication is used for the subject injury/illness but also for a second ratable condition, then it should be counted only once because the interferences of ADLs and/or side effects accrue only once. For example, if a pain medication is used for a herniated lumbar disc and also for chronic pain from a rotator cuff injury, then the medication is only counted once.

3. Each month is considered to contain 28 days. For a medication to be considered as being taken for 1 month, it must be taken for at least 21 days during the month. If not, then it is considered to be an as-needed medication and the number of points accrued is the number of days divided by 28, which is then applied to the points applicable for the medication. For example, if an individual used a medication to treat the nausea caused by migraine headaches 7 d/mo, on the average, and that medication was used once a day and inserted rectally, then the total number of points would be:

    a. The points for rectal administration once a day times 25% (7 d/mo or 7/28 equals 25%)

4. Medications used to treat side effects of a medication used to treat the subject incident/injury are also covered. For example, if potassium supplementation is used to

prevent hypokalemia in an individual taking a diuretic for job-related hypertension, then this medication is also counted in the BOTC. The exceptions to this rule are:

a. If the alleged medication side effect cannot be supported by the medical literature

b. If the alleged medication side effect cannot be supported by the medical records

c. If the alleged medication side effect is rated separately, in conjunction with an alternative and/or more appropriate organ system injury/illness

d. If the so-called medication is a nonprescription/alternative medication that is not prescribed by an osteopathic or allopathic physician

5. For as-needed medications, the average frequency per month is used. For example, if a medication is used once a day, 7 d/mo, then the factor of 25% would apply, as seen in the example earlier. In contrast, if that medication were given 3 times a day, 7 d/mo on an as-needed basis, that would represent a 75% factor.

6. Rules are found for dietary modifications.

7. Rules are found for assigning points for specific procedures.

The BOTC assigns points for frequency and routes of administration of medications (tables B-2a and B-2b), routes of administration (table B-2c), dietary modifications (B-3), and procedures (B-4). Table B-1 translates the accumulated points into a whole-person impairment rating.[6(pp607,608)]

In general, the impairment rating created by BOTC is combined with the impairment rating for the subject incident. However, each chapter should be reviewed for specific uses and information.

CASE EXAMPLES
Example 1: Peripheral Vascular Disease

Ms Smith is a 56-year-old woman who sustained a crush injury to her right lower leg. She had no orthopedic injuries and she was treated conservatively. However, she developed extensive thromboses in the right calf, extending into the popliteal system. She was treated with anticoagulants. After 6 months, she was taken off the anticoagulants but developed recurrent thrombosis. Since that time, she has had recurrent peripheral edema in the right lower extremity that required elastic supports for control. She has been maintained, indefinitely, on anticoagulants. What is her impairment rating?

Using table 4-12[6(p69)], she merits class 1 impairment of the lower extremity for peripheral vascular disease because of the persistent edema controlled by elastic supports. Her impairment rating for that condition is 2% of the lower extremity. Table 9-3[6(p186)] describes supplemental impairment based on the BOTC for various hematological issues. Using this table, she has an additional 5% impairment of the whole person based on the chronic anticoagulant therapy.

Example 2: Diabetes Mellitus

Mr White and Mr Black both have type 2 diabetes mellitus. Both are 54 years old and are 170 cm tall. However, Mr White weighs 78 kg (BMI = 27.0) and Mr Black weighs 138 kg (BMI = 47.8). Mr White "watches his diet" and takes metformin twice a day. He sees his physician 4 times a year for diabetic checkups. His hemoglobin A1c (HbA_{1c}) has averaged 6.4% (normal, <6.5%) over the past 2 years. In contrast, Mr Black is on a restrictive diet. His diabetes has been treated for the past 12 months. Originally, he weighed 154 kg (BMI, 53.3). He tries to adhere to a calorie limit of 1500 calories per day with fish at least twice a week and the bulk of his calories coming in the form of healthy carbohydrates. He is supposed to eat 3 times per day with a snack in the evening. He takes metformin twice a day, insulin glargine once a day, and a short-acting insulin before each meal (4 times a day). He adjusts his premeal insulin according to his blood sugar and anticipated caloric intake. Thus, he checks his blood sugar level 4 times a day. He sees his physician monthly for nutritional advice, blood sugar monitoring, and periodic HbA1c levels. Bariatric surgery and psychiatric counseling are being considered. He also sees a dietitian once a month. His HbA_{1c} has averaged 10.4% over the past 6 months.

What is the impairment rating for each of these individuals?
Both individuals have type II diabetes. This can be rated as a static condition using the sixth edition of the AMA guides.[6] Using table 10-10 on page 234, Mr White most closely fits class 1 impairment by meeting the following criteria:

- Presence of diabetes and/or metabolic syndrome established biochemically, treated with a relatively simple single oral medication and/or dietary regimen; no insulin use
- Normal HbA_{1c} 0.06 to 0.065 (6%–6.5%)
- BOTC: 1 to 5 points

This accrues 1% to 5% impairment of whole person. His BOTC points were calculated using section 10.1f[6(pp217,218)] of the endocrinology chapter (chapter 10, The Endocrine System). For taking a single medication, twice a day, he received 2 procedure-based impairment points and 2 points for dietary modifications, minimal. His total BOTC points were 4, fulfilling the last bulleted point needed for inclusion in class 1 impairment.

Mr Black's BOTC points were calculated in the following manner:

- For taking parenteral medications more than twice a day, he received 5 points.
- For severe dietary modifications, he received 10 points.
- For monitoring his blood sugars 4 times per day, he received 4 points.
- When added, he had 19 points.
- He qualified for class 4 impairment by meeting the following criteria: Presence of diabetes, established biochemically, that is not consistently controlled despite use of any treatment regimen and adherence to an aggressive dietary and medication regimen; documented by abnormal glucose measurements
- Increased HbA_{1c} greater than 0.10 (>10%)
- BOTC: greater than or equal to 16 points

This calculation accrues 16% to 28% impairment of the whole person. Note that he received no additional impairment for the frequency of his medical encounters. This aspect of his rating is subsumed into overall impairment rating.

Example 3: Myelodysplastic Syndrome

Mr Green is a 54-year-old man who developed a myelodysplastic syndrome as a result of benzene exposure on his job. Fatigue and weight loss 1 year ago led to a diagnosis of progressive anemia. A bone marrow examination disclosed myelodysplasia with excessive blasts. He received combination chemotherapy for 4 months followed by an allogeneic hematopoietic cell transplant. His condition was stable and at maximum medical improvement 6 months following the transplant. However, he did not achieve a complete response and had persistent anemia. He was unresponsive to erythropoietin and required a transfusion of packed red blood cells every 6 to 8 weeks. His hemoglobin counts hovered between 7.5 and 9.7 g/dL. What is his impairment rating?

Using table 9-5,[6(p189)] he qualifies for class 2 impairment for anemia based on meeting the following criteria:

- History of chronic anemia with continuous mild symptoms and occasional moderate exacerbations or occasional transfusions required
- Hemoglobin greater than or equal to 8 g/dL but less than 10 g/dL

Higher classes require more symptoms and more frequent transfusions. He has 11% impairment of the whole person. In addition, he receives impairment based on issues related to the BOTC. He has had 4 cycles of chemotherapy; using table 9-3,[6(p186)] each cycle accrues 1% impairment of whole person (total 4%). Because of the bone marrow transplant, he qualified for 10% impairment of whole person. In addition, averaging 1 transfusion every 2 months for the past 6 months, there is an additional 3% impairment of the whole person. His impairment rating is 11% + 4% + 10% + 3% = 28% impairment of whole person.

SUMMARY

All editions of the AMA guides traditionally rate impairment based on static deviations from population or personal norms in addition to rating based on interferences in ADLs. The BOTC method of impairment rating assists in overcoming difficulties when rating internal medicine conditions, when normative metrics may be lacking and impact on ADLs are not readily determined. With the changes in the sixth edition of the AMA guides, the BOTC model has been adapted to provide alternative operational metrics for functional losses associated with these conditions.

ACKNOWLEDGMENTS

The BOTC is a concept that originated out of a need for rating medical impairment for a variety of internal medicine conditions and was initially conceived and developed by the American Medical Association for the sixth edition of the AMA guides.[6]

REFERENCES

1. American Medical Association. Guides to the evaluation of permanent impairment. 4th edition. Chicago: American Medical Association; 1993.
2. Altman PL, Gibson JF Jr, Wang CC. Handbook of respiration. Dayton (OH): Wright-Patterson AFB; 1958.
3. American Heart Association Science Advisory. Assessment of functional capacity in clinical and research application. Circulation 2000;102:1591.
4. McArdle WD, Katch FI, Katch VL. Exercise physiology: energy, nutrition, and human performance. Philadelphia: Lea & Febiger; 1981.
5. Passmore R, Durnin JVGA. Human energy expenditure. Physiol Rev 1955;35:801.
6. Rondinelli RD, editor. Guides to the evaluation of permanent impairment. 6th edition. Chicago: AMA Press; 2008.

Measuring Quality of Life Loss in Litigation

Patricia A. Murphy, PhD, MS, BA

KEYWORDS

- Institute of Medicine model • Veterans Affairs • World Health Organization
- WHOQOL-100 • WHOQOL-BREF • Computer adaptive testing
- Patient-centered care

KEY POINTS

- The complexity challenge in QOL assessment is more easily addressed since the advent of computer adaptive testing (CAT), which is used by physicians and rehabilitationists in the administration of psychometric instruments to determine QOL loss.
- It is now possible to write algorithms to capture QOL data through text-mining.
- If QOL domains and their factors could be accessed through text-mining, it would make for an extraordinary opportunity for much needed doctoral level research in QOL issues for injured workers in workers' compensation programs.

INTRODUCTION

The Institute of Medicine (IOM) model[1] was derived directly from Nagi, who defined disability as "a function of the interaction of the person with the environment." In this model, physical and social environmental risk factors (and biologic and lifestyle risk factors) were described as independent variables that exist at all stages of the process. These factors affect progression within the model, and their control therefore affects (prevents) disability. Although the IOM model is highly respected for its explanation of disability, it has some limitations. Under the first IOM model, "impairment is defined as a discrete loss or abnormality, mental, physical, or in 1997 an IOM report added two important concepts to the Disablement Model: the concepts of secondary conditions and quality of life."[2] The IOM model describes quality of life (QOL) "affects and is affected by the outcomes of each stage of the disabling process. Within the disabling process, each stage interacts with an individual's quality of life."

Secondary conditions are defined as "any additional physical or mental health condition that occurs as a result of having a primary disabling condition."[3] Secondary

In Memory of John M. Williams 1947–2005.
The author has nothing to disclose.
Department of Women & Gender Studies, University of Toledo, 2801 W. Bancroft Street, MS 965, Toledo, OH 43606-3390, USA
E-mail address: patricia.murphy2@utoledo.edu

conditions are "related to a primary health condition and atypical or premature aging with disabilities are important because they can affect physical and psychological functioning, independence, and participation in community life; including work. They can diminish quality of life…"[3]

For example, a female student of mine, in her fifties, with cerebral palsy had never had a mammogram for two reasons. First, her disability was perceived by caregivers and medical professionals as a static condition, and so there was no need for care other than her primary disability care issues. Although she was most likely experiencing premature aging in her fifties, no attention was paid to the need to examine possible secondary conditions, such as breast cancer, which commonly occurs in later life. Second, the mammogram facility was not set up for a person who used a wheelchair and who could not stand. Therefore, it was not possible for my student to have a mammogram. My student started coughing. She died 2 weeks later with advanced breast cancer. My student had reached out to participate in the newly developed Disability Studies Program at the University of Toledo. The courses were designed for access by the disability community and the able student community. The courses had enriched her QOL by increasing her social interactions, which was then destroyed by the development of a secondary condition.

In contrast, "comorbidities are health conditions that develop independently of the primary condition." Comorbidity is addressed later in this article, but one study revealed that in workers' compensation cases, the three major comorbid conditions are obesity, diabetes, and opioid addiction.[4–8]

The Veterans' Affairs Schedule for Rating Disabilities includes QOL or health-related QOL assessment.[9] The complexities of the Veterans Affairs systems for rating and scoring QOL exceed the limits of this article.

Independent medical evaluations (IMEs) are conducted to determine if an individual who has acquired a disability, injury, or illness is eligible for benefits. In addition to the customary assessment tools in IME practice, there is also a demand that QOL measurements be used. As Gibbons and colleagues[10] point out: "Increasing priority placed on patient centered care reflects a long-standing movement toward patient-centered metrics and away from sole reliance on disease-centered measures of severity, impact, and burden." Patient-centered metrics are found in the QOL psychometric instruments described later.

Developments in computer adaptive testing (CAT) allow for ease in administering WHOQOL-BREF as contrasted to paper and pencil testing. Gibbons notes that "computational techniques could make patient-reported outcome and experience measures less time-consuming while making them more accurate, relevant, useful, and interesting." As we enter the era of big data, the demand for CAT will increase. This is a significant development for IME physicians, whose time and ready access to such outcome information is otherwise limited.

Unfortunately, research leading to the development of psychometric instruments, which are reliable and valid, to address QOL in workers' compensation systems, Social Security Disability Insurance, and personal injury cases has not kept pace with the development of instruments measuring QOL as it pertains to illness and disease.

No effort has been made to precisely score the loss of QOL in the cases described in this article, because the scoring method is complex and beyond the scope of this discussion. It is now possible to Google the WHOQOL instruments and download them. Obtaining the scoring manual must be done through the World Health Organization (WHO) to convert the raw scores to transformed scores. Instructions for scoring can also be found online.

In 1999, my coauthor and I argued in our book[11] that "rehabilitationists, by training and experience, are in the best position to provide a multi-dimensional perspective on the impact of impairment, disability and/or other traumatic life events." All case histories described here resulted from my role as a vocational rehabilitation counselor in California, Nevada, and New Mexico providing services in more than 1000 afflicted persons in workers' compensation programs and personal injury lawsuits. In contrast, my experience in providing services in Social Security Administration (SSA) hearings was limited to less than five cases.

SOCIAL SECURITY ADMINISTRATION AND THE NEED FOR A QUALITY OF LIFE ASSESSMENT

The Social Security Act defines disability as the inability to engage in any substantial gainful activity by reason of a medically determinable physical or mental impairment that is expected to result in death or is expected to last for a continuous period of not less than 12 months. This definition "is at odds with most contemporary thought about the concept of disability and is in itself a barrier to the SSA work disability revision process."[2] Jette[2] notes that "conceptual confusion is a particular barrier to the improvement of the SSA process for determining eligibility for Social Security Disability Insurance and Supplemental Security Income related to work disability."

In 2013, a group of researchers[12,13] developed CAT for SSA disability determination. CAT, in their study, would be used to assess physical function, which is one of the domains in the WHOQOL-BREF. CAT is already used in the administration of the WHOQOL-BREF. CAT may enable the systematic and formal assessment of QOL metrics in an effective and time-efficient manner to warrant their inclusion on a routine basis going forward (See Alan M. Jette and colleagues' article, "The Work Disability Functional Assessment Battery (WD-FAB)," in this issue for an example of how this may work.)

EXAMPLES OF WHOQOL-BREF ASSESSMENT IN PERSONAL INJURY CASES

Personal injury cases, such as injuries sustained in automobile accidents, are where the least restrictions on providing QOL assessment are found. All case histories reported here come from my background as a vocational rehabilitation counselor.

Case 1

Mr A was a 33-year-old developmentally impaired individual with cerebral palsy. He used a wheelchair and lived in a group home. Mr A had joined the Person First Movement, which demanded that persons with mental retardation be seen as persons first and not by their diagnosis. When Mr A attended a Person First conference, he roomed with another group member. This other man was much larger than Mr A and, unfortunately, sexually assaulted him. When Mr A complained, he was dismissed from the group home and ended up on the streets of Denver with his alcoholic mother. The perpetrator remained in the group home. Mr A was subsequently diagnosed with post-traumatic stress disorder (PTSD).

The physical domain

Mr A had a preexisting condition of cerebral palsy that necessitated his use of a wheelchair. Therefore, his mobility was already impaired before the sexual assault. Without the wheelchair, Mr A had to crawl on his hands and knees. Although the goal of group homes is to foster independence in their residents, little effort had ever been made to assist Mr A with this goal. Realistically, there were few jobs open to Mr A because of his preexisting conditions.

The psychological domain
In addition to mobility issues, Mr A's cerebral palsy left him intellectually disabled. Mr A had a diagnosis of PTSD as a result of the sexual assault. The result was negative feelings and loss of self-esteem. One manifestation of this condition was his anger with the Person First Movement. "They are just using me," he said.

The social relationships domain
Mr A's personal relationships meant that he had to not only deal with his alcoholic mother on the streets of Denver, but also lost his friends in the group home. His social support provided by the group home counselors was also destroyed. He could not return to the group home because the perpetrator was still there. Because of his negative associations with the Person First Movement as result of the attack during the conference, he lost the relationships he had and would have developed in the organization.

The environment domain
Mr A's safety and security were severely compromised because of his created homelessness. His financial situation was destroyed because he could not receive his Social Security benefits without an address. His health was at risk because of homelessness, which brings little access to good nutrition, cleanliness, and adequate sleep. Transportation was problematic because of his use of a wheelchair and the lack of buses that could provide wheelchair service. This meant he could not get to welfare offices to apply for assistance. Survival became Mr A's goal and leisure time and obtaining information necessary for a QOL were denied to him.

Outcome
A lawsuit was filed against the group home and against the perpetrator. The case went to a jury trial. The QOL assessment allowed the jury to realize how every aspect of Mr A's life had been impacted by the sexual assault. The group home was obliged to make a financial settlement. This allowed Mr A to find a smaller group home with only two other residents in the home. He was able to purchase a computer and printer, so he could have some social contacts via the Internet. His Social Security Disability Insurance benefits were restored. Settlement income was set up to be disbursed on as-needed basis. The QOL assessment used the scoring system provided by WHO and resulted in a 70% loss of QOL. Mr A clung to his dignity even when he had to get down from his wheelchair and crawl to the witness box during the jury trial. In fact, Mr A asserted himself and made the decision to get into the witness box even though he could have stayed in his wheelchair to testify. Mr A had an impressive dignity and sense of self despite his life challenges.

Case 2

Mr D was an older gentleman, retired from his work as a sales manager. He led a full life as a golfer, hiker, and companion to his wife of many years. Because of an automobile accident, he sustained a fracture to his hip that never healed correctly. The result was an inability to play golf, hike, or make love to his wife without a great deal of pain. Driving was also difficult.

The physical domain
Mr D experienced pain while walking, driving, and having sexual relations with his wife. His mobility was impaired because of the hip fracture. His normal routine and activities

were restricted by his physical limitations. He had to take pain medication on a regular basis. Because Mr D was retired, work capacity was not considered in the analysis. Mr D's life expectancy may also have been shortened because hip fractures in the elderly are often lethal.

The psychological domain

Mr D's body image was damaged. Before the accident, he considered himself an active older gentleman. Loss of self-esteem or seeing himself now as a crippled elderly man, which is a stereotype about the aging body, had no place in his life before the accident.

The social relationships domain

Mr D's relationship with his wife was impaired because he no longer enjoyed sexual relations with her because of his hip pain. His companionship with his fellow golfers and hikers was further limited because of his pain, negatively impacting his ability to develop and maintain new relationships and friends.

The environment domain

Mr D's hip fracture meant that he was no longer as safe and secure as he was before the accident because he was now perceived as elderly and feeble. His active physical leisure time was severely curtailed. Because driving was painful, his ability to transport himself on errands and long trips was difficult.

Outcome

A lawsuit was filed against the insurance company whose driver was at fault for the accident. Because QOL determinations were not readily accepted in New Mexico until 1998, the defense attorney in this personal injury case was able to convince the jury that the QOL assessment was irrelevant. Mr D received only the amount of fees he would have paid to play golf twice per week for 10 years. The issue of a shortened life expectancy caused by the potential lethality of hip fractures in the elderly was also ignored.

Case 3

Ms G was a 25-year-old married woman with two children. Both she and her husband worked and her income was needed by the family. Before an automobile accident, Ms G held a clerical position in a local real estate firm. Driving to work one morning, a beam used in highway construction tore loose and came through the windshield of her automobile and hit her dominant arm, rendering not only her arm, but her hand useless. The result was a diagnosis of PTSD and of a flail arm. Because Ms G was taking her children to school that day, her PTSD was compounded by the children's trauma. All were afraid to even get into an automobile let alone drive or ride in an automobile.

The physical domain

Ms G experienced a loss of energy, sleep was difficult because of the adjustment she had to make with her flail arm, and her mobility was severely compromised because she was now a one-handed person in terms of function. This, in turn, meant activities of daily living, such as dressing, bathing, and grooming, were all impaired. She lost her job as a clerical worker because she could no longer use a computer keyboard.

The psychological domain

Ms G had negative feelings about her body and her body image. Her self-esteem was damaged. Her PTSD experience was amplified by the PTSD her two children also acquired as a result of the accident. She reached out to her God by attending church but spiritual comfort eluded her because of the PTSD and the failure of her God to cure her flail arm. Ms G now doubted her competence in every area of her life. It is not unusual for people who acquire a disability as an adult to assume that their problem-solving abilities have also been damaged.

The social relationships domain

Any social support Ms G might have gained from family and friends was tainted by them telling her she was "lucky because she hadn't died." Because of her damaged body and damaged body image Ms G was reluctant to make love with her husband thereby eroding her personal intimacy with her husband. Her fear of driving a car or even being in a car meant that visiting friends or looking for a job was difficult. Her relationship with her children was now problematic because her children expressed their PTSD through anger at her for not protecting them. All of the societal prejudice experienced by people with disabilities was now shared by Ms G.

The environment domain

Ms G's safety and security were compromised because of her disability. Having only one functional arm and hand meant she could not do such things as opening a car door while holding keys or a purse or groceries. This meant that she would be vulnerable in parking lots and would most likely not be able to defend herself from a potential assailant (women with disabilities are two times more likely to be assaulted than able-bodied women). Her functionality within the home environment was compromised in terms of cooking, holding pans, taking a chicken out of the oven, and reaching up into the family kitchen cupboards. The family's financial situation was strained by her loss of income from her job. Leisure activities, such as picnics with her children, swimming, and dancing with her husband, were greatly reduced because of lost income and physical capabilities. Transportation became a highly problematic issue and her husband had to drive the family members everywhere.

Outcome

After Ms G's attorneys were able to use the QOL assessment to settle the case and prevent the need for a trial, Ms G was able to address the many needs in her life after the accident. Ms G obtained counseling for herself and her family regarding her PTSD and for assistance in developing a new functioning and healthy family dynamic. She obtained training in driving as a one-handed person and counseling for her and her children about being in a car and being in a car driven by their mother. Ms G was able to purchase a one-handed computer keyboard for the left hand. After training on this keyboard, she was able to start a job search as a clerical worker. The job search was not easy because of prejudice against people with disabilities. She had to take a job at less pay than she received from her former job. After referral to occupational therapy, Ms G obtained kitchen utensils, such as a grip and grab tool to get dishes from high cupboards and tools for ease in handling pots and pans. Methods for dressing, buttoning shirts and trousers, and putting on sock and shoes all helped Ms G in recapturing normalcy and regaining functional independence with her daily life activities. All of these rehabilitative services and products were provided at the expense of the insurance company and did not include the settlement for the loss of QOL in this young mother's life.

WORKERS' COMPENSATION PROGRAMS AND QUALITY OF LIFE ASSESSMENT

Formal QOL assessments are presently not routinely included in workers' compensation claims assessments and the exclusion of thorough and systematically collected data of this kind may inadvertently and negatively impact an injured worker's ability to receive the full benefits to which they are otherwise entitled.

Routine addition of QOL assessments may be misperceived as a costly and unnecessary additional administrative burden. Despite this, Big Data may make it possible for an ease in administering the WHOQOL-BREF and other psychometric instruments. In addition, workers' compensation programs are storing workers' compensation claims data at such a rate that workers' compensation data warehouses have been created. Analysis of these storehouses of data becomes possible through various methodologies, particularly text-mining.

One expert calls for the use of this data to "build predictive models focused on the underlying costs that increase claim severity."[14–17] This risk management expert notes that

> Generally, today's predictive models include the following fields: age, gender, cause of injury, nature of the injury, work status and job classification. To create better predictive modeling tools, organizations should increase the categories of data they capture, perhaps including: prescribed medications (specifically narcotics), socioeconomic factors (such as education level), psycho-social factors (such as job satisfaction) and distance to the primary worksite.[14]

In my opinion, Transue[14] is calling for a QOL assessment. With the development of the WHOQOL-100 and the WHOQOL-BREF, there are categories and key words used in text-mining of the previously overwhelming and unrecognized data, which might lead to improvements in injury prevention, recommendations for better medical treatment, higher rates of successful return to work outcomes, and reduction in costs. Lewis[18,19] reveals that predictive analytics reduces costs in workers' compensation programs from 4% to 15%.

Such QOL assessments would address comorbid conditions that increase workers' compensation medical costs and most likely complicate case management and rehabilitative efforts.[20] According to a study sponsored by The Hartford,[4] the three major comorbid conditions are obesity, diabetes, and opioid addiction. This study used text-mining of a million cases to ferret out the conditions that increased claims costs. This, in turn, allowed The Hartford to make recommendations to employers for preventive measures thereby reducing medical costs overall and to get a clearer understanding of the needs of injured workers with comorbid conditions.

I argue that vocational rehabilitation counselors have always collected all the data for each injured worker as needed for a QOL analysis but not in a coherent manner as described in the WHOQOL-BREF examples previously. Without the concept of QOL or the permission to use such an analysis, the vocational rehabilitation counselor has often been stuck with unused or unreported information about the situation of the injured worker. For example, a sanitation worker with an injury to his lower back surprised me when he told me that from time to time, he still visited his truck even though it was an old truck and was on its way to the junk yard to be crushed. I did not put this in any report but what I learned from this injured worker was that there was more to his case than covering the medical costs of his injury, providing subsistence income until the injury is resolved, and return to his previous employment or new employment.

There is a profound loss here. The loss of identity as a worker should not be underestimated. Along with that loss, there is disengagement with fellow workers, adjustment with family who find the injured worker at home disrupting the patterns of family life, the loss of income, and the humiliation of being suspected as faking it by the employer and the insurance carrier.

Recognition of these losses makes for a better understanding of the needs and behaviors of injured workers, potentially leading to better outcomes for injured workers in the workers' compensation process.

DISCUSSION

The advantage of administering the WHOQOL-BREF and other psychometric instruments measuring QOL includes allowing for deeper insight into the impact of how injury and disease changes an individual's life in any given case. When an injured worker visits his truck, we learn that an industrial injury is more than medical treatment, legal issues, rehabilitation issues, and financial concerns.

The disadvantage lies in the time it takes to administer the WHOQOL-BREF. CAT may solve this problem. However, there will be patients who are not able to use this method and such patients will require assistance in answering the questions in the WHOQOL-BREF.

If scoring of the WHOQOL-BREF is not completed using CAT, then sending the completed WHOQOL-BREF to the WHO for scoring will be required. Time delays in using the completed instrument will occur.

Theoretically, physicians could use the WHOQOL-BREF in their practices particularly if CAT is added to the methods of creating and completing medical records. However, there is something lost in setting down a patient in front of a computer to complete the WHOQOL-BREF rather than a face to face administration of the instrument. For example, a patient who is in denial about the extent of his/her injury may respond to the question "Do you worry about your pain or discomfort?" by selecting 1 (not at all) on the 5-point Likert scale for each question. Such a response could elicit further inquiry. For example, in one workers' compensation case, the injured worker counted on his fellow union workers to assist him in his 2 years to retirement as a commercial painter. Other than medical treatment, he shrugged off other benefits. He wanted to return to work despite having fallen and broken bones in both feet.

In workers' compensation programs, rehabilitation counselors and rehabilitationists are the professionals who go to the worker's home for the initial evaluation. A home visit is often more revealing than any psychometric instrument. Furthermore, the rehabilitationist reviews medical records; conducts labor market surveys; refers patients to work evaluation centers; and administers various psychometric instruments, such as interest inventories, aptitude testing, and the WHOQOL-BREF or other QOL instruments. The rehabilitationist also places workers in training programs, on the job training arrangements, and workplace accommodations while monitoring the worker on his/her path to return to work. In short, no other professionals are likely to spend as much time with the worker as do rehabilitationists. It is rehabilitationists who should administer the WHOQOL-BREF.

SUMMARY

"The quality of life approach or paradigm adds complexity to the discussion of damages in litigation, but it also adds accuracy."[11,21] The complexity challenge in QOL assessment is more easily addressed since the advent of CAT, which can be used by physicians and rehabilitationists in the administration of psychometric instruments to determine QOL loss.

It is now possible to write algorithms to capture QOL data through text-mining. For example, the WHOQOL-BREF provides the terminology via its four domains of QOL: (1) physical, (2) psychological, (3) social, and (4) environmental. The factors within the domains can also be captured[22,23]:

- The physical domain: pain, energy, sleep, mobility, activities, medication, and work
- The psychological domain: cognitions, positive feelings, self-esteem, body image, negative feelings, and spirituality
- The social relationships domain: interpersonal relations, sexual relations, and social support
- The environment domain: safety and security, home environment, finance, health/social care, information, leisure, physical environment, and transportation.

If the Hartford Insurance Company can text-mine a million workers' compensation cases to discover comorbid conditions, then QOL domains and their factors can also be accessed through text-mining. This would provide an extraordinary opportunity for much needed doctoral level research in QOL issues for injured workers in workers' compensation programs.

REFERENCES

1. Brandt EN Jr, Pope AM, editors. Institute of Medicine (US) Committee on Assessing Rehabilitation Science and Engineering. Washington, DC: National Academies Press (US); 1997.
2. Jette A. Conceptual issues in the measurement of work disability. Washington, DC: The National Academies Press; 2000.
3. Lankasky K. Secondary conditions and aging with disability. Washington, DC: National Academy of Sciences; 2007.
4. Advisen Insurance Intelligence. Mining workers' compensation data nets valuable cost-control gems. The Hartford; 2014.
5. A 21st century system for evaluating veterans for disability benefits. Chapter 3: impairment, disability, and quality of life. Washington, DC: The National Academies Press; 2007.
6. The critical need to reform workers' compensation. Washington, DC: American Public Health Association; 2017. Policy Number: 2017. Available at: https://www.apha.org/policies-and-advocacy/public-health-policy-statement.
7. Cobb CW. Measurement tools and the quality of life. San Francisco (CA): Redefining progress; 2000.
8. Diaz PA, Schwarzbold ML, Thais ME, et al. Psychiatric disorders and health-related quality of life after severe traumatic brain injury: a prospective study. J Neurotrauma 2012;29(6):1029–37.
9. Veterans Affairs Schedule for Rating Disabilities. Available at: https://www.benefits.va.gov/WARMS/bookc.asp. 2017
10. Gibbons C, Bower P, Lovell K, et al. Electronic quality of life assessment using computer-adaptive testing. J Med Internet Res 2016;18(9):e240.
11. Murphy PA, Williams JM. Assessment of rehabilitative and quality of life issues in litigation. Boca Raton (FL): CRC Press; 1999.
12. Pengsheng N, McDonough CM, Jette AM, et al. Development of a computer-adaptive physical function instrument for Social Security Administration disability determination. Arch Phys Med Rehabil 2013;94(9):1661–9.

13. Post WM. Definitions of quality of life: what has happened and how to move on. Top Spinal Cord Inj Rehabil 2014;20(3):167–80.
14. Transue B. Improving workers' comp starts with improving your data 2012. Available at: http://www.rmmagazine.com. Accessed February 2018.
15. Tulsky DS, Kisla PA, Victorson D, et al. Overview of spinal cord injury-quality of life (SCI-QOL) measurement system. J Spinal Cord Med 2015;38(3):257–69.
16. WHO. Field trial WHOQOL-100. Geneva (Switzerland): Division of Mental Health, World Health Organization; 1995.
17. WHO. WHOQOL: measuring quality of life. Geneva (Switzerland): Division of Mental Health, World Health Organization; 1997.
18. Lewis RT. Using data and analytics in workers' compensation. Available at: http://www.verisk.com. Accessed January 17, 2018.
19. Meeberg GA. Quality of life: a concept analysis. J Adv Nurs 1993;18:32–8.
20. Robinette B. The impact of comorbid conditions on workers' compensation medical costs. Workcomp Wire 2010.
21. Pawlowska-Cyprysiak K, Konarska M, Zolnierczyk-Zreda D. Self-perceived quality of life of people with physical disabilities and labour force participation. Int J Occup Saf Ergon 2013;19(2):185–94.
22. Skevington SM, Lofty M, O'Connell KA. The World Health Organization's WHOQOL-BREF quality of life assessment: psychometric properties and results of the international field trial. A report from the WHOQOL group. Qual Life Res 2004;13:299–310.
23. Thompson HM, Reisner SL, VanKim N, et al. Quality-of-life measurement: assessing the WHOQOL-BREF scale in a sample of high-risk transgender women in San Francisco, California. Int J Transgend 2015;16(1):36–48.

Determination of Medicolegal Causation

J. Mark Melhorn, MD[a,b],*, Marjorie Eskay-Auerbach, MD, JD[c]

KEYWORDS

- Causation • Risk • Worker's compensation • Law • Science • Assessment

KEY POINTS

- Causation determinations are complex.
- Science is required for appropriate causation determination.
- NIOSH/ACOEM/AMA methodology is key to scientific approach to causation.
- Hill criteria assist in assessing quality of science.
- Workers' compensation and personal injury cases require both a medical and legal causation determination.

INTRODUCTION

Determining causation has been and continues to be a critical issue for diagnosis and treatment of medical conditions and diseases. Although the science of causation continues to improve with additional research, its definition remains elusive. Why? Because the concept of causation has different meanings and applications for various parties and, therefore, the establishment of causation can be elusive in some situations.

By definition, cause is something that results in an effect. In philosophy, if A causes B, then A must always be followed by B. In science, physicians and statisticians use statistics to arrive at suggestions from observational studies that A probably caused B. Biostatistics can never establish exact cause and effect but gives the probability that A contributed to B. This is because of the multiple additional factors that may directly or indirectly have also contributed to or allowed increased risk for the

No commercial or financial conflicts of interest.

Funding support provided by The Hand Center. Dr J. Mark Melhorn grants Elsevier the right to print and reproduce this material but retains the right to use this material in future work products with appropriate acknowledgment of this source.

[a] The Hand Center, 625 North Carriage Parkway, Suite 125, Wichita, KS 67208-4510, USA;
[b] Department of Orthopaedics, University of Kansas School of Medicine – Wichita, Wichita, KS, USA; [c] SpineCare & Forensic Medicine, PLLC, 5610 East Grant Road, Tucson, AZ 85712, USA
* Corresponding author. The Hand Center, 625 North Carriage Parkway, Suite 125, Wichita, KS 67208-4510.
E-mail address: melhorn@onemain.com

individual. For example, smoking cigarettes may contribute to lung cancer, but ciga-rette smoking itself does not always cause lung cancer in every individual who smokes because lung cancer is also linked to other environmental exposures (risk factors) and to the health of the individual (nonoccupational risk factors).

In law, causation considers 2 separate and distinct components: cause in fact and proximate (or legal) cause. Furthermore, the legal threshold for cause in fact ("but for") varies by jurisdiction. Proximate cause is the legal question if the 2 events are so closely linked that liability should be attached to the first event for producing the sec-ond event, the harm.

PREVALENT PERCEPTIONS OF WORK-RELATEDNESS

Opinions regarding causation should be based upon the current best available scien-tific evidence. Occasionally, opinions about causation are offered based on popular opinion despite scientific evidence to the contrary. For example, the speculation that carpal tunnel syndrome is related to keyboard use is widely accepted, but un-proven. Because this proposed linkage is appealing and pervasive and seems to make sense, the lay press has advanced this association despite several quality sci-entific investigations that have found little or no relationship between carpal tunnel syndrome and keyboard use.[1–4] This promotion by the nonmedical media actually rep-resents a form of publication bias.[5] However, this does not mean that future quality studies will not establish a relationship; medicine has been wrong in the past and it will likely be wrong in the future.[6] Therefore, the process of determining whether a symptom, injury, or illness is factually and legally due to employment conditions is important to the individual patient (employee), the employer, and other workers who may be exposed to similar conditions.

This has led to the concept of the current workers' compensation system as a medi-cally driven legal compromise, commonly described as the "Grand Bargain" between labor and employers.

> Workers' Compensation is a very important field of law, if not the most important. It touches more lives than any other field of the law. It involves the payments of huge sums of money. The welfare of human beings, the success of business, and the pocketbooks of consumers are affected daily by it.
> —Judge E.R. Mills, Singletary v Mangham Construction, 418 So.2d 1138 (Fla. 1st DCA 1982).

MEDICAL CAUSATION VERSUS LEGAL CAUSATION

Work-relatedness and/or accident-relatedness, in the context of industrial and/or per-sonal injuries, involves concepts of medical and legal causation. The two may be mutually exclusive. Definitions of medical causation and legal causation arise from different sources—one from science and the other from the desire for social justice. For physicians treating injured workers, understanding the differences between the two concepts is essential, as outlined in **Boxes 1** and **2**.[7]

Medical causation deals with scientific cause and effect. For example, a physician may conclude, based on well-accepted principles of science, that exposure A in a workplace is likely to have caused B. In a different example that includes ambiguity or inconsistency in the test results, the physician may conclude that A did not cause B. In both cases, the physicians made cause-and-effect determinations that were based solely on scientific principles. Presumably, any challenge to that physician's conclusions would similarly be rooted in science.

> **Box 1**
> **Medical causation**
>
> Evidence slowly accumulates over time, with criticism of published studies leading to better designed studies with lower risk of bias
>
> Eventually a CONCLUSION is so probable it becomes generally accepted as Scientific Truth
>
> *Data from* Melhorn JM. The method for causation analysis - upper limb. In: 19th Annual AAOS Workers' compensation and musculoskeletal injuries: improving outcomes with back-to-work, legal and administrative strategies, edited by J.M. Melhorn. Rosemont, IL: American Academy of Orthopaedic Surgeons, 2017.

Legal causation is dealt with in the courts from which our system of justice developed. The courts do not have their origins in science, and therefore the laws they developed were historically, not scientifically, derived. The medieval courts were, in part, institutions of the church, and their function was to promulgate, not to discern order. Laws applying to causation have 3 origins: common law, also known as case law, which is developed by judges through decisions of courts; statutes that are adopted through the legislative process; and regulations issued by the executive branch.[6]

Modern medical science accepts that events of nature, including medical conditions, are multifactorial, and as such are more likely to be controlled by the laws of probability than by a single cause. Yet, in law, finding the causal connection between a wrongful act and harm is essential to assigning legal responsibility. As Judge Kirby observed in Chappel v Hart (1998) 195 CLR 232; [1998] HCA 55 [87], both civil law and common law courts have searched for principles to provide a filter to eliminate those consequences of the defendant's conduct for which he [or she] should not be held liable. The search sets one on a path of reasoning which is inescapably complex, difficult and controversial. The outcome is a branch of the law which is highly discretionary and unpredictable. Needless to say, this causes dissatisfaction to litigants, anguish for their advisers, uncertainty for judges, agitation among commentators and friction between healthcare professionals and their legal counterparts.[8]

There may always be a chasm between science and the courts, that is, between why things are and how things ought to be. It should not come as a surprise, therefore, that causation in law is not the same as in science.[6]

Does proximate cause (the legal question) affect the medical opinion of causation? Is it important for a physician to understand proximate cause? Most physicians who are called on to testify concerning medical issues in personal injury litigation do not

> **Box 2**
> **Legal causation**
>
> May occur before the TRUTH is known
>
> Experts TESTIFY that A causes B
>
> Opinions [conclusions] accepted as "Evidence"
>
> But may later be proven as FALSE
>
> *Data from* Melhorn JM. The method for causation analysis - upper limb. In: 19th Annual AAOS Workers' compensation and musculoskeletal injuries: improving outcomes with back-to-work, legal and administrative strategies, edited by J.M. Melhorn. Rosemont, IL: American Academy of Orthopaedic Surgeons, 2017.

understand that judges and attorneys view "causation" quite differently than do members of the medical community. For example, medical practitioners tend to be concerned with all possible causes of the patient's current medical condition, whereas legal practitioners in personal injury cases generally focus on a particular event as possibly precipitating, hastening, or aggravating a particular aspect of the patient's condition to the extent that the event in question is, in legal language, the "proximate cause" of an injurious event and therefore establishes the possibility of assigning blame. Furthermore, proximate cause is often established by previous court causes. Specifically, the physician must understand the legal threshold for determining a "legal causation link" when providing their opinion.

OCCUPATIONAL FACTORS AND NONOCCUPATIONAL FACTORS

Although by definition work-related disorders affect workers, the disorder may not necessarily have been caused or significantly aggravated by work.[9] To determine occupational cause or association for a risk factor, the evaluator must consider both the individual and the workplace.[10]

What is risk? Risk is the probability that an event will occur. In epidemiology, it is most often used to express the probability that a particular outcome will follow a particular exposure. A risk factor can be an environmental, behavioral, or biological factor confirmed by temporal sequence, ideally in prospective, longitudinal studies, that if present directly increases the probability a disease will occur, and if absent or removed reduces that probability as outlined in Hill criteria in **Box 4**.[6] Risk factors are part of the causal pathway or the causal model, whereby the individual can be exposed to multiple factors.[11]

Precisely which factors predominate in the etiology of work-related medical conditions is the subject of ongoing debate. Often a specific diagnosis has a multifactorial etiology (occupational and nonoccupational) and a single cause cannot be identified.[11] Furthermore, the impact of the medical diagnosis on the individual is significantly affected by the role of biopsychosocial factors.[12,13] The concept of biopsychosocial factors has been expanded to include the economic impact of the diagnosis on the individual and is described as "biopsychosocioeconomic" factors.[14]

Individual risk factors for the development of disability from biological stimuli include age, gender, and inherited health characteristics. Risk factors associated with psychosocial and/or biosocial issues are depression, current substance abuse, somatoform pain disorders, longer duration of symptoms, higher association of anxiety disorders, higher levels of stress in life events, lower levels of lifestyle organization (goal directedness, performance focus and efficiency, timeliness of task completion, and organization of physical space), and coping skills or strategies.[15] Additional biopsychosocioeconomic risk factors include previously learned behavior, less time on the job, more surgeries, a higher frequency of acute antecedent trauma, indeterminate musculoskeletal diagnoses, self-reported higher pain levels, more anger with their employer, a greater psychological response or reactivity to pain, a strong sense of entitlement, and/or having an attorney and being involved in litigation with their employer.[16,17]

WHY A PROCESS TO DETERMINE CAUSATION IS IMPORTANT

So how does the physician scientist opine regarding causation in a specific individual? Again, it is important to understand that the legal system has established 2 levels of "scientific evidence" for the courts. These levels were established by 2 cases commonly known as Frye and Daubert. The courts base their decisions on evidence that has been deemed worthy of being admitted into the records of their proceedings. Not all evidence is admissible. Rules of evidence are intended to help ensure that the foundation on which the court's decisions regarding the disputes is appropriate. In addition, assuring fairness when opposing or conflicting scientific opinions are involved is often not a simple matter.

Frye (1923) in general says "...in admitting expert testimony deduced from a well-recognized scientific principle or discovery, the thing from which the deduction is made must be sufficiently established to have gained general acceptance in the particular field to which it belongs." Viewed analytically, the *Frye* court placed the ultimate locus of control of admissibility not in the courts but in the scientific community.[6] At the core of this decision was the contention that judges should defer to scientific experts; "general acceptance" was sufficient for a properly qualified expert to testify.[18]

Daubert (1992) changed the trial courts' focus from whether the expert's opinion was consistent with scientific consensus or "general acceptance" to whether the expert's techniques and methodology were valid.[18]

In general, under Daubert, we [the judges] must engage in a difficult, two-part analysis. First, we must determine nothing less than whether the experts' testimony reflects 'scientific knowledge,' whether their findings are 'derived by the scientific method,' and whether their work product amounts to 'good science.'...Second, we must ensure that the proposed expert testimony is 'relevant to the task at hand,'...that is, that it logically advances a material aspect of the proposing party's case.[6]

Essentially, Daubert established the judiciary as the gatekeeper for expert testimony, with the requirement that judges find as a preliminary fact that the methods and principles underlying expert testimony are sufficiently valid to support that testimony. Four factors have been identified for the court to consider when making that determination. Included in evaluating the scientific validity of expert testimony is whether the research "has been subjected to peer review and publication."[19]

Efforts to disqualify experts on the basis of their failure to comport with Daubert are not uncommon, and courts are more frequently using Daubert hearings to closely examine the reliability of expert witness opinions. Therefore, is it incumbent on the physician scientist to present expert testimony that is "good science" and "relevant"? This can consistently be accomplished by using the method developed by the National Institute for Occupational Safety and Health (NIOSH), the American College of Occupational and Environmental Medicine (ACOEM), and the American Medical Association (AMA) Causation ("blue book").[20]

NATIONAL INSTITUTE FOR OCCUPATIONAL SAFETY AND HEALTH/AMERICAN COLLEGE OF OCCUPATIONAL AND ENVIRONMENTAL MEDICINE/AMERICAN MEDICAL ASSOCIATION METHOD FOR DETERMINATION OF WORK-RELATEDNESS

In January of 1979, *A Guide to The Work-Relatedness of Disease*,[21] which outlined the methodology in **Box 3** (see also Table 3-2 in Hegmann and colleagues[20]), was published by the US Department of Health, Education, and Welfare, Public Health Services, Centers for Disease Control, and NIOSH. Each of these 6 steps requires the application of Hill criteria as outlined in **Box 4** (see also Table 3-2 in Hegmann and colleagues[20]).

Of the Hill criteria, temporality, strength of association, consistency, and dose-response relationship are considered the most important. Experimental evidence, coherence, specificity, analogy, and plausibility are considered relatively weak criteria. Without 1 of the first 4 criteria satisfied, meeting only 1 or more of the other criteria is

---

Box 3

National Institute for Occupational Safety and Health/American College of Occupational and Environmental Medicine steps for the determination of work-relatedness of a disease

1. Identify evidence of disease

2. Review and assess the available epidemiologic evidence for a causal relationship

3. Obtain and assess the evidence of exposure

4. Consider other relevant factors

5. Judge the validity of testimony

6. Form conclusions about the work-relatedness of the disease in the person undergoing evaluation

Adapted from Kusnetz and Hutchinson, eds. DHEW, CDC NIOSH, Pub. No. PB298-561, 1979 and Occupational medicine practice guidelines, 2nd and 3rd editions. ACOEM OEM Press, 2004, 2008, 2011; with permission.

---

consistent with weak evidence and can only be considered as suggesting a hypothesis that will require further study.[20] It is not always necessary or appropriate to apply all of the Hill criteria to each of the steps used to determine work-relatedness or injury-relatedness.

Some courts have also established an additional requirement of a relative risk greater than 2.0.[6,20] Relative risk compares the outcome if the risk factor is present with the outcome if the risk factor is not present, and is calculated by dividing the risk in the former group by the risk in the latter group.

Step 1 requires an appropriate medical diagnosis of the condition in question.

Step 2. Once the diagnosis is confirmed, a literature search is performed to determine the current best science. If the diagnosis is included in the AMA Causation blue book, this step has already been completed for the evaluator.[22] If the diagnosis is not included in the AMA Causation blue book it may be possible to use a similar diagnosis

---

Box 4

Assess the studies using the updated Hill criteria; apply the criteria to individual studies (especially a–c) and the studies as a whole (a–l)

a. Temporality

b. Strength of association

c. Dose-response relationship

d. Consistency

e. Coherence

f. Specificity

g. Plausibility

h. Reversibility

i. Prevention/elimination

j. Experiment

k. Analogy

l. Predictive performance

for the analysis. Lacking the ability to complete Step 2 with these options, the AMA Causation blue book provides a specific method for scoring the studies obtained during the literature search and determining a level of evidence.[23]

It is important to remember that evidence is not the same as proof; the purpose of scoring studies is to determine whether evidence is weak and therefore not convincing, or strong. Studies vary with respect to internal validity and external validity or practical usability, which may affect their score (https://www.cebma.org/faq/what-are-the-levels-of-evidence/). Randomized controlled trials (RCTs) are designed to yield the lowest chance of bias and the highest internal validity, and are often considered the gold standard. Cohort studies and other observational studies have lower internal validity (https://www.cebma.org/faq/what-are-the-levels-of-evidence/); however, they are administratively easier to conduct and less expensive than RCTs. The highest-quality evidence may not exist for a given clinical issue; however, critical assessment of the available research facilitates finding the best current evidence.

Step 3. Assessing evidence of exposure is where Hill criteria are applied to the epidemiologically identified risk/association factors and then to whether the individual experienced a sufficient exposure to the risk/association factor to be considered an appropriate exposure for this specific individual.

Step 4. Other relevant factors are sometimes overlooked but are potentially very important. This takes into consideration who the individual is. In other words, do they have individual risk factors (nonoccupational) that overshadow possible occupational risk factors in the development of their diagnosis?

Step 5. Judge the validity of the science. This requires applying the appropriate Hill criteria to the individual case, and the quality of the science (study design pyramid; **Fig. 1**).[20] The study design pyramid may be used to rank the relative value of various

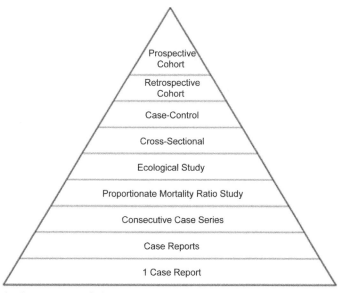

Fig. 1. Study design pyramid. (*From* Hegmann KT, Thiese MS, Oostema SJ, Melhorn JM. Causal associations and determination of work-relatedness. In: Guides to the evaluation of disease and injury causation, edited by J.M. Melhorn, J.B. Talmage, W.E. Ackerman, and M.H. Hyman. Chicago, IL: American Medical Association, 2013, p. 105–114; with permission.)

types of study designs. In general, the prospective cohort study is the strongest epidemiologic study design for most exposures and is assumed to have better characteristics than the other designs. However, the hierarchy of studies in the design pyramid is not absolute because it is possible to have a poorly conducted cohort study but a well-conducted case-control study.[20] Thus, the need to apply the steps in AMA Causation blue book Chapter 4, "Methodology." In general, high-quality studies allow the expert to testify to a greater degree of certainty.

Step 6. Form conclusions. The final step is the overall assessment of whether a causal association is likely to exist. Because this step requires substantial judgment, it also requires that the person(s) evaluating the body of evidence make(s) statements of how sure they are that there is or is not a causal association. Workers' compensation systems generally require that a physician's opinions or conclusions regarding causation be expressed in terms of probability that a given condition has or has not arisen in the course and scope of employment (ie, is or is not work-related) to a reasonable degree of medical certainty.[20] Although each jurisdiction may have unique wording, other considerations would include: a probability greater than 50% standard; preponderance of the evidence; or reasonable degree of medical probability.[20] The courts usually prefer that such opinions be expressed in terms such as more likely than not.

EXAMPLE

Providing a causation analysis that includes scientific support for the opinions rendered in an occupational or personal injury report/evaluation will generally meet the criteria set forth in Daubert (not all the criteria need to be met and will depend on the specialty). As discussed earlier, the quality of the literature cited is important; it is possible to find some literature that will support any opinion. The definition of evidence-based medicine refers to the best evidence available. A sound causation analysis using critically assessed high-quality literature will likely withstand a lawyer's scrutiny.

As a brief example, consider a 55-year-old, 250-lb kindergarten teacher, who reported the onset of left knee pain after climbing up and down a small stepladder repetitively to hang her students' mobiles from the ceiling. At one point she fell off the ladder, twisting her left knee. She noticed swelling of the left knee at the end of the day, with some deep aching pain, and reported her condition to the principal. She was referred to an occupational medical clinic for treatment, and after a course of nonsteroidal anti-inflammatories, physical therapy, and injections, continued to have pain. An MRI scan of the left knee was obtained and demonstrated a medial meniscal tear and mild cartilage thinning at the patellar apex and lateral patellar facet with thinning of the cartilage in the medial compartment. The claim was accepted as work-related and she underwent arthroscopic surgery.

Six weeks after surgery, she reports the onset of right knee pain and attributes that to increased weight bearing on the right while recovering from her left knee procedure. Her physical therapist has endorsed this explanation for her new complaints, based on the patient's reported functional loss of the left knee, which may represent an impairment. The *AMA Guides to the Evaluation of Permanent Impairment* (6th edition) defines impairment as "a significant deviation, loss, or loss of use of any body structure or function in an individual with a health condition, disorder, or disease." An MRI scan of the right knee shows some degenerative changes, with chondromalacia of the patella and thinning of the cartilage in the medial compartment. You are asked to determine whether the right knee complaints are related to the initial left knee injury (which was accepted as work-related).

Using the recommended methodology for assessing causation, the following factors would be considered:

1. Diagnosis: right knee pain with mild-to-moderate degenerative changes of the knee.
2. Exposure: did an injury occur in this individual? Are postoperative gait changes a plausible cause of injury to the right knee?
3. Epidemiology: does the available medical literature identify an association between an abnormal gait after surgery and disorder in the unoperated knee?
4. Other relevant factors: are there known risk factors, such as age and weight, that more likely account for degenerative changes in the knee?
5. Validity: Are there conflicting data with respect to the information obtained, or are they reliable?
6. Evaluation and conclusions.

This is an example whereby "it is only common sense" that surgery on the left knee would result in increased weight bearing on the right and pain from an aggravation of underlying degenerative joint changes. However, a search of the literature (AMA Causation blue book) produces no quality evidence-based medical literature supporting such a relationship.[24] Other relevant factors that more likely explain MRI findings include age and weight.[25] The presence of bilateral disease is consistent with age-related changes.[25] The conclusion can be drawn, to a reasonable degree of medical probability, that surgery on the left knee was not the cause of the right-sided knee pain.

SUMMARY

The determination of causation has become the gateway to treatment and reimbursement in workers' compensation and a method to determine the impact of proximate cause in personal injury cases. The science of causation is constantly evolving, which is improving our understanding of individual physical thresholds, associated risk factors, and individual biopsychosocioeconomic factors. New laws place constantly changing legal thresholds for determining work-relatedness and proximate cause. The underlying foundation for fairness is quality science to support decisions made by the legal system to provide injured workers with the appropriate treatment to restore their function and decrease their functional impairment and/or assist in determining appropriate proximate cause in personal injury cases.

REFERENCES

1. Szabo RM. Appendix B. Dissent. Musculoskeletal disorders and the workplace: low back and upper extremities. Washington, DC: The National Academies; 2001. p. 439–57.
2. Melhorn JM, Martin DP, Brooks CN, et al. Upper Limb. In: Melhorn JM, Talmage JB, Ackerman WE, et al, editors. Guides to the evaluation of disease and injury causation. 2nd edition. Chicago: American Medical Association; 2013. p. 243–356.
3. Nathan PA, Meadows KD, Istvan JA. Predictors of carpal tunnel syndrome: an 11-year study of industrial workers. J Hand Surg Am 2002;27A:644–51.
4. Andersen JH, Thomsen JF, Overgaard E, et al. Computer use and carpal tunnel syndrome: a 1-year follow-up study. JAMA 2003;289:2963–9.
5. Melhorn JM. Epidemiology of musculoskeletal disorders and workplace factors. In: Mayer TG, Gatchel RJ, Polatin PB, editors. Occupational musculoskeletal

disorders function, outcomes, and evidence. Philadelphia: Lippincott, Williams & Wilkins; 1999. p. 225–66.

6. Melhorn JM, Ackerman WE, Glass LS, et al. Understanding work-relatedness. In: Melhorn JM, Talmage JB, Ackerman WE, et al, editors. Guides to the evaluation of disease and injury causation. 2nd edition. Chicago: American Medical Association; 2013. p. 15–104.

7. Melhorn JM. The method for causation analysis—upper limb. In: Melhorn JM, editor. 19th Annual AAOS workers' compensation and musculoskeletal injuries: improving outcomes with back-to-work, legal and administrative strategies. Rosemont (IL): American Academy of Orthopaedic Surgeons; 2017.

8. Freckelton I, Mendelson D. Causation in law and medicine. Burlington (VT): Ashgate Publishing; 2002.

9. Chapell RW, Bruening W, Mitchell MD, et al. Diagnosis and treatment of worker-related musculoskeletal disorders of the upper extremity. Evidence Report/Technology Assessment Number 62. Rockville (MD): Agency for Healthcare Research and Quality; 2003.

10. Melhorn JM. Work injuries: the history of CTD/RSI in the workplace. In: Melhorn JM, Zeppieri JP, editors. Workers' compensation case management: a multidisciplinary perspective. Rosemont (IL): American Academy of Orthopaedic Surgeons; 1999. p. 221–50.

11. Talmage JB, Melhorn JM. A physician's guide to return to work. Chicago: AMA Press; 2005.

12. Melhorn JM, Kennedy EM. Musculoskeletal disorders, disability, and return-to-work: repetitive strain. the quest for objectivity. In: Schultz IZ, Gatchel RJ, editors. Handbook of complex occupational disability claims: early risk identification, intervention and prevention. New York: Springer; 2005. p. 231–54.

13. Melhorn JM. Occupational orthopaedics. J Bone Joint Surg Am 2000;82A:902–4.

14. Melhorn JM. Negotiation—the art of communication regarding Dx, Tx, causation, and outcome. In: Melhorn JM, Barr JS Jr, editors. 17th Annual AAOS workers' compensation and musculoskeletal injuries: improving outcomes with back-to-work, legal and administrative strategies. Rosemont (IL): American Academy of Orthopaedic Surgeons; 2015.

15. Melhorn JM. Disability upper extremity. In: Schmidt RF, Willis WD, editors. Encyclopedia of pain. 2nd edition. New York: Springer; 2013.

16. Himmelstein JS, Feuerstein M, Stanek EJ, et al. Work related upper extremity disorders and work disability: clinical and psychosocial presentation. J Occup Environ Med 1995;37:1278–86.

17. Sikorski JM, Molan RR, Askin GN. Orthopaedic basis for occupationally related arm and neck pain. Aust N Z J Surg 1989;59:471–8.

18. Gatowski SI, Dobbin SA, Richardson JT, et al. Asking the gatekeepers: a national survey of judges on judging expert evidence in a post-Daubert world. Law Hum Behav 2001;25:433–58.

19. Faigman DL. The *Daubert* revolution and the birth of modernity: managing scientific evidence in the age of science. Davis Law Review 2013;46:893–930.

20. Hegmann KT, Thiese MS, Oostema SJ, et al. Causal associations and determination of work-relatedness. In: Melhorn JM, Talmage JB, Ackerman WE, et al, editors. Guides to the evaluation of disease and injury causation. 2nd edition. Chicago: American Medical Association; 2013. p. 105–14.

21. Kusnetz S, Hutchison MK, editors. A guide to the work relatedness of disease (revised). DHEW (NIOSH) publication No. 79-116. Washington, DC: U.S. Department of Health, Education, and Welfare; 1979.

22. Melhorn JM, Talmage JB, Ackerman WE, et al. Guides to the evaluation of disease and injury causation. 2nd editiob. Chicago: American Medical Association; 2014.
23. Shields NN, Fetter DA, Dietz MJ, et al. Lower limb. In: Melhorn JM, Talmage JB, Ackerman WE, et al, editors. Guides to the evaluation of disease and injury causation. 2nd edition. Chicago: American Medical Association; 2013. p. 357–88.
24. Brigham CR, Brooks CN, Talmage JB. Evaluating causation for the opposite lower limb. In: Melhorn JM, Talmage JB, Ackerman WE, et al, editors. Guides to the evaluation of disease and injury causation. 2nd edition. Chicago: American Medical Association; 2013. p. 769–74.
25. Liu TC, Leung N, Edwards L, et al. Patients older than 40 years with unilateral occupational claims for new shoulder and knee symptoms have bilateral MRI changes. Clin Orthop Relat Res 2017;475(10):2360–5.

Life Expectancy Expert Reports

Common Mistakes and Appropriate Process

Pierre J. Vachon, PhD, MPH, LLM, Esq

KEYWORDS

• Life expectancy • Evidence • Expert witness • Expert report • FRE 702

KEY POINTS

- Examining life expectancy opinions via the prism of evidentiary standards confers tangible benefits to the observer.
- This simple heuristic, although far from having perfect sensitivity, can highlight faults in the analysis, be they failure of qualification, methods, or facts.
- It can be useful for a witness tasked with producing a life expectancy opinion to keep in mind the commandments of the law as to the sufficiency of an opinion.
- Abiding by the requirements in a transparent fashion can not only ensure that the opinion will be deemed admissible, but also increases the likelihood that the opinion will be properly understood and appreciated by the finder of fact.

INTRODUCTION

Detailed technical explanations exist to show the process of elaborating a life expectancy opinion.[1,2] The purpose of this article is to illustrate some common mistakes in life expectancy opinions, and contrast those with appropriate tools and approaches. This will be done by addressing legal and technical aspects of life expectancy expertise, with the dual goal of helping potential experts avoid common pitfalls and helping consumers of life expectancy opinions, be they legal actors or witnesses to other aspects of the legal case, assess the quality and soundness of life expectancy expertise.

To guide this exercise, the article starts by considering the legal foundation. The admissibility of expert witness testimony in US Federal Courts is governed by Rule 702 of the Federal Rules of Evidence[3]: "A witness who is qualified as an expert by knowledge, skill, experience, training, or education may testify in the form of an opinion or otherwise if:

a. The expert's scientific, technical, or other specialized knowledge will help the trier of fact to understand the evidence or to determine a fact in issue;

The author has no commercial of financial conflict of interest.
Life Expectancy Consulting, 129 Holly Terrace, Sunnyvale, CA 94086, USA
E-mail address: vachon@lifeexpectancyexpert.net

Phys Med Rehabil Clin N Am 30 (2019) 611–619
https://doi.org/10.1016/j.pmr.2019.03.008   **pmr.theclinics.com**
1047-9651/19/© 2019 Elsevier Inc. All rights reserved.

b. The testimony is based on sufficient facts or data;
c. The testimony is the product of reliable principles and methods; and
d. The expert has reliably applied the principles and methods to the facts of the case."

The admissibility of evidence is a matter of law, and therefore decided by the judge. In the case of expert testimony, judges act as gatekeepers to preclude the admission of testimony that would be confusing, incorrect, or improper, among other aspects. It is an essential role of the court to analyze and assess the validity of expert testimony in light of evidentiary rules.

In considering the ways a report can go wrong, the author will relate to this rule, and especially to sections (c) and (d), as they relate to the most common mistakes observed. It should be pointed out that this rule does not apply in all forensic instances in the United States, but the main alternative – the Frye rule[a] – is broadly similar in most of its applications. Furthermore, other jurisdictions outside the United States often employ standards one would not consider too dissimilar to Rule 702. For example, Civil Procedure Rule 53.03 of Ontario[4] requires that a report comprise, among other things the expert's reasons for his or her opinion, including,

A description of the factual assumptions on which the opinion is based
A description of any research conducted by the expert that led him or her to form the opinion
A list of every document, if any, relied on by the expert in forming the opinion

Although no pretense will be made that vast volumes of jurisprudence can be summed up in a convenient and perfectly accurate maxim, it is not unreasonable to employ a somewhat shorthand version of these standards, stated as: a qualified expert applies standard and accepted methods to appropriate facts. The author will thus in turn consider each of those aspects, for good and bad.

QUALIFIED EXPERT

There is no clear bright-line rule that identifies the threshold one needs to cross to qualify as an expert. The corpus of jurisprudence on the issue of course offers some guidance, but a large number of somewhat but not always consistent legal opinions hardly constitutes a line. This is probably why many purported experts claim the status on the grounds of the very words mentioned in FRE 702: "education, training and experience"[b]. This may be fair and appropriate in large fields of study or specialties. For instance, one might claim expertise in biochemistry by pointing to a graduate degree in that precise field and to concrete laboratory work. In the case of life expectancy, no such degrees or routinely performed practicum exists. It could thus be appropriate to ask what qualifies one to claim expert status. It is probably not fair to reduce expertise in life expectancy to a singular academic path or type of practice and experience, but one can nonetheless

---

[a] *Frye v. United States*, 293 F. 1013 (D.C. Cir. 1923). This decision was superseded at the federal level by Daubert v. Merrell Dow Pharmaceuticals, 509 U.S. 579 (1983). Many states still use the Frye standard, however, so the expert should verify what the standard is in the relevant jurisdiction.

[b] Few claim qualification by skill, perhaps because it would seem somewhat circular to claim that one should be considered an expert at a skill because one has skill.

identify some elements that probably should be considered. To explore what those could be, one needs to consider what life expectancy actually is, and is not.

The very term expectancy signifies that the sought quantity is an average[c]. That this requires pointing out seems strange, but several alleged experts seem to confuse or conflate average and median[d]. The reports of such experts usually comprise an excuse masquerading as a justification, relying in part on the following: in the civil law context in the United States, there exists an evidentiary standard where acceptance of a claim by the fact finder requires that the claim be more likely than not. Ergo, providing the median survival time is the appropriate way of addressing the issue before the court. This justification is silly. If a party was preoccupied with that question, he or she would ask it directly, by requesting an opinion on the median survival time. This is a distinct quantity from life expectancy, with its own uses and purposes[e]. Any purported expert who conflates median survival time with life expectancy is either per se incompetent or unwilling to abide by the request of a party. This alone would be disqualifying.

Considering this, one can probably safely postulate as a necessary precondition that any expert on life expectancy should have some formal training in statistics, sufficient to know the difference between mean and median. This of course is a minimalist baseline that should be used more to exclude those not meeting it than qualify those who do. The bar for sufficient qualification may be more narrowly qualified by supplementing this baseline with a requirement that the claimed expert be knowledgeable of standard life expectancy concepts such as mortality rates[f] and life tables, and be adept at using and applying such concepts. Familiarity with such may usually be gained by academic work in statistics, biostatistics, epidemiology, demography, or actuarial science. It is likely that a standard medical curriculum would not discuss or teach the methodological tools employed to calculate life expectancy. It would follow then that such a curriculum would not, by itself, qualify the ordinary physician or clinician as an expert on life expectancy under rule FRE 702 (a).

It should also be pointed that out that extensive experience in dispensing improper opinions on life expectancy cannot be leveraged into qualifying experience under FRE 702. Or, put another way, "I've been doing wrong for a long time" cannot be used to support the conclusion that "therefore, I qualify as an expert." It should also be patently obvious that the routine or casual treatment of patients with a given condition, no matter how extensive or frequent, does not make one an expert on life expectancy with that given condition. That this is so, for both methodological and mathematical reasons, is explained in the next section.

---

[c] Life expectancy can be defined as the expected (or average) remaining years of life for a group or individual.

[d] The average is the sum of all observations divided by the number of observations: $\{(x_1 + x_2 + \ldots + x_n)/n\}$. The median would be the middle observation of a sorted array of values; for n sorted values of x_i, the median would be $x_{n/2}$. For a numerical example, consider that the mean of the values $\{1, 1, 2, 11, 25\}$ is 8, while the median is 2 (the middle value being the third of 5 observations).

[e] For instance, answering a possibly legally significant question such as whether a given person was more likely than not to survive an additional 10 years absent an accidental death.

[f] Which are distinct from a probability of death. Not knowing the difference should also count as a disqualifier. A succinct illustration: if 100 individuals are alive at the beginning of the year, and 12 die during the year, the probability of death is $12/100 = 0.12$, whereas the mortality rate (presuming a uniform distribution of deaths in the interval) would be $12/(100-(12/2)) = 12/94 \approx 0.1276$.

STANDARD AND ACCEPTED METHODS

There should be no need to explain that a proper opinion, sufficient to qualify for admissibility under the rules, cannot be founded solely on feelings or subjective impressions. Yet, I have seen too many reports where the substance of the opinion was set on no more a foundation than a vocal assertion of education, training, and experience. An opinion, to meet the standards of admissibility under FRE 702 (c), should explain the process that leads to the opinion with sufficient detail that it be intelligible to and reproducible by another qualified expert. One should remember the mantra of just about all high school math teachers: "you need to show your work."

This standard allows one to immediately recognize that some alleged methods are in fact not methods at all. Statements containing the word experience are usually a clue that the witness is about to declare a value without evidentiary support. Such proclamations often take the form of "I've seen countless patients with this condition, and they live to normal ages." Absent systematic and well-ordered data collection protocols, citations to one's personal experience are misguided[g]. This can be inferred from basic calculations on the life expectancy of a 10-year old girl in the United States. The general population life expectancy would be 71.9[h] (to an age of 81.9). An excess risk[i] (in the mortality rate) of 1 death per 1000 population for age 10 to the end of the life course gives a life expectancy of 69.3 years (to an age of 79.3 years). An excess of 2 deaths per 1000 population gives a life expectancy 66.8 years (to an age of 76.8 years). The number of observations one would require to properly assess whether the excess risk is 1, or 2, or 0 deaths per 1000 population is not within the ambit of any practicing physician. Proper values for mortality cannot be gleaned from casual ongoing observation; they must emanate from well-designed studies of suitably large populations, with proper tracking and follow-up. Any purported method comprising casual observation as an element necessarily fails under FRE 702 (c).

Another common attempt at methodology is to default to normal without inquiry or justification. This often takes the form of "sure, the patient suffers from condition X, but with good care, there should be no reduction in life expectancy"[j]. It should be clear that this is usually not the product of the application of any method. Such a statement should only result from a thorough search of the literature sufficient to support a finding of absence of evidence, and not from mere clinical introspection. Similarly, the invocation of good care as an absolute guard against hazards cannot be asserted without supporting, empirically substantial

---

[g] For example, there can be slight yet statistically meaningful dissimilarities in severity of disease, or there can be improper record keeping or loss of patients in follow-up, other biases common in epidemiologic studies like self-selection, or any other of countless problems that dedicated epidemiologists try to fight in large systematic studies, and often fail to completely counteract. A casual physician's observation cannot reach the precision required for proper, quantitative inference.

[h] Based on the latest mortality rates from the Human Mortality Databases,[5] U.S. 1x1 table.

[i] Excess death rate (EDR) can be defined as the absolute difference between the mortality rate of the general population and that of the afflicted population. For example, if the mortality rate at a given age of the general population is 0.022 and the corresponding age-specific mortality rate for the afflicted population is 0.0245, the EDR for that condition at that age would be 0.0245–0.022 = 0.0025.

[j] Another not rare enough claim is the pseudo-technical expression 'near normal'. This one is particularly insidious in that it simultaneously concedes a departure from normality yet also ascribes no value to the divergence, undoubtedly to appear accommodating, all the while suggesting that the magnitude of the value is small enough as to not merit quantification. To say that the life expectancy is normal despite no evidence might be lazy and somewhat incompetent, but to say it is near normal is to perpetrate a purposeful and calculated deception on the finder of fact.

evidence. This common trope seems to tap in the perception that medical practice is adept at fending off routine and ordinary complications, such that no measurable effect on mortality can be discerned. This is contrary to reality. Conditions as commonplace and undramatic as hypertension are associated with higher than baseline mortality. If the patient can be ascribed to a given population (eg, the population of people who suffer from hypertension), then, the mortality of that population should be ascribed to the patient, ceteris paribus[k].

There exists another all too common attempt at estimation that, sadly, still needs to be refuted and denounced. Many reports have postulated that a given condition is associated with a certain decrease of x years in life expectancy. This is incorrect for several reasons, but one can merely point out that life expectancy is not the result of simple linear calculations. If it is true that the condition is associated with a life expectancy smaller than the general population by a value of x at a given age y, the same condition at age y+5 would not be associated with a difference of x. The size of the difference would vary with age. For example, a condition associated with a difference of 3.0 years of life expectancy for a 40-year-old Canadian man may be associated with a difference of only 2.5 years for a 65-year-old US woman. This fact is obvious enough – and mathematically demonstrable – that any report claiming such a constant absolute reduction should be discarded on the grounds of failure to qualify under FRE 702 (c), and on the grounds that the witness does not qualify as an expert under FRE 702 (a), for lack of understanding of how life expectancy functions.

The fact that life expectancy does not operate in a linear fashion also precludes the application of what in other contexts might be deemed appropriate methods. If the life expectancy of a person with a given condition is known for some ages but not all[l], one cannot simply fit a linear regression model to estimate at other ages. This would be somewhat akin to estimating the accrued value of a sum subject to compound interest by linearly extrapolating. This can be illustrated with actual values. If one consider the life expectancy of a U.S. man[m] aged 20 years (LE = 57.4) and aged 40 years (LE = 38.8), a linear extrapolation would yield an estimate for age 60 of 20.2. The true value is in fact 21.8. This divergence may seem somewhat small, but it is nonetheless a significant departure from the true value. If this is not enough to convince everyone of the absurdity of this so-called method, one only needs to consider that projecting still onward for age 80 yields a life expectancy estimate of 1.6, when the true value is 8.5, and the projected value at 90 would be -7.7, a mathematical impossibility. Linear extrapolation therefore cannot be considered a valid method under FRE 702 (c) for any significant interval.

Similarly, interpolation based on a linear approach to mortality rates can also lead to incorrect results. Applying a constant excess mortality rate of 1 death per 1000 population for the whole life course would make the life expectancy at birth of a US female 55.1 years. Applying 2 deaths per 1000 population makes it 39.6 years. Instinct may suggest that applying 1.5 deaths per 1000 population would yield a life expectancy of 47.35 years (the average of 39.6 and 55.1 years), but the actual value is in fact

---

[k] Unless of course, sufficient studies can be produced to show that a good care/bad care divide exists and yields statistically significant disparities in survival.

[l] for example, if it is known that the life expectancy at age 20 is 30.5, and the life expectancy at age 30 is 26. It is possible that the life expectancy at other ages is not known directly; estimations would then be required.

[m] All values based on Human Mortality Database mortality rates.

46.4 years. An expert opinion should therefore shun linear interpolation or extrapolation over any substantial time interval[n].

In contrast to this brief review of some bad methods or nonmethods, one can point to a collection of generally accepted standard methods that one could and should expect to see incorporated in a life expectancy opinion. The basic methods are well known[o] and broadly accepted across several related academic fields – and have been for quite some time.[6]

A life expectancy is the product of the application of mortality rates[p] over the life course of the patient. The goal of this application is to measure the probability of survival from the given age to the end of an entire life course, often truncated at 100[q]. As explained in the technical publications cited previously, this is almost always performed with a life table.

The basic input of a life table is a set of mortality rates. It is common practice to build a life table using general population rates (eg, US mortality rates for the general population) and adjusting the risk in light of the profile of the individual. This can be done by incorporating excess mortality rates (adding an absolute number to the base rates) or applying multipliers (relative risks or mortality ratios, which multiply the base rates)[r]. The soundness of each approach depends on context, but both are recognized as valid tools when used properly. In the case of multiple conditions, it may be required for the expert to apply both methods simultaneously, such as when 2 independent risks[s] are associated with multiplicative risks, and the ultimate, total risk would be the sum of the relative risks[t].

---

[n] Interpolation over intervals of 1 year are still incorrect, but the deviation from a proper model is usually small enough as to not significantly affect ultimate results. Most published life tables incorporate some linear approximation for such small intervals. Special care and alternate methods may be warranted for very low and very high ages.

[o] It is not unreasonable to summarize the steps to creating a life expectancy report as follows: 1) identify the characteristics of the individual of interest that correlate to higher or lower than average mortality, 2) find reliable source materials to determine the levels of mortality associated with each condition (taking into account age and severity), 3) calculate the difference in mortality rates (either an EDR, or a Mortality Ratio) associated with the condition compared with the general population, 4) extrapolate as required those differences in mortality rates to get a complete series of mortality rates (from the age of the individual to the terminal age of the life table [eg, from the given age to 100]), 5) apply standard life table methods to calculate a probability of survival to each age and ultimately, generate a life expectancy value.

[p] Or probability of death, provided one uses the appropriate calculations.

[q] This is arbitrary. Appropriateness of the terminal age, whether 100 or 110 or 120, depends on the desired sensitivity and available information. For most cases, rounding out the table at age 100 will have no significant effect on the ultimate value.

[r] See again, for instance, Singer[1] or Vachon & Sestier[2]; for actual relative risks or excess death rates, see for example, Brackenridge, Croxson & Mackenzie.[7]

[s] In an ideal world, one would manage to always find reliable information on the exact profile. Both publications most often relate to a single condition. To calculate the life expectancy of an individual suffering from 2 distinct conditions, one cannot rely on the hope that a given publication address the risk associated with both conditions simultaneously. It will in most cases be necessary to consider each risk independently and ascribe both to the individual by combining the risk under assumptions that need to be disclosed to the fact finder (eg, risks are independent and additive, or multiplicative, or supermultiplicative …).

[t] Condition A could be associated with a relative risk of 1.5 and condition B with a relative risk of 2.5. The total risk, if the components are independent, would be the base risk plus the excess risks of (1.5–1) = 0.5, and (2.5–1) = 1.5, for a total of 1 + 0.5 + 1.5 = 3. Or, in an alternative notation, +50 and + 150 sum up to +200. That would correspond to an input series of mortality rates all 3 times the value of the mortality rates of the general population.

When the expert finds relevant mortality rates[u], odds will be that the data only capture a partial age range. Studies rarely yield mortality data for advanced ages, both because of sample size issues and costs of extended follow-up. But as has been mentioned, life expectancy is an average, and a valid calculation requires mortality rates for the entire age range (up to the end of the life table). This conundrum will usually be resolved by employing standard, mathematically sound extrapolation methods[8] in conjunction with the identified mortality rates to build a complete series of mortality rates tailored to the individual's conditions for the entire lifespan. This in turn allows for the application of standard life table methods to produce life expectancy.

One can conclude thus that a reliable and qualified opinion on life expectancy will make use of standard, accepted methods, free of personal introspection, and disclosed and explained by the author in such a way as to allow for replication and critical evaluation by fellow qualified experts. Appropriate methods cannot include techniques that could lead to aberrant results or techniques relying implicitly or explicitly on linearity.

APPROPRIATE FACTS

Facts, in the context of a life expectancy opinion, can relate to 2 distinct areas: facts about the patient, and facts about the science of the conditions at play. Facts about the patient are usually gleaned from medical reports[v]. Given this, it is unlikely that a life expectancy expert would dispute medical facts. In the case of ambiguity, the safest course of action is probably to leave determination to the trier of fact and offer alternative opinions based on the different possibilities. For example, it would be appropriate for an expert to present a report stating that "if it is found the patient suffered from condition y, the life expectancy is x_1, but if it is found otherwise, the life expectancy is x_2." For the life expectancy expert to attempt posing a diagnosis might constitute a violation of FRE 702 (a), or (b), or (d).

Facts pertaining to the science are much more the purview of the expert. By science, the author here means the actual, prevailing levels of mortality associated with the conditions present (eg, what is the actual mortality rate associated with treated hypertension of between 140 and 160). Absent direct access to large amounts of high quality data, ascertaining mortality rates requires making use of already processed data, be it in the form of published studies, dedicated monographies, or statistical agency data[w]. In such contexts, the expert is at least 1 step removed from the raw data and will have to exercise some judgment to evaluate the relevance and trustworthiness of the data.

For this, reliance on a single source of data (a singular study) is counterindicated. It is of course possible that a given source could be the best and most accurate. But publication bias and biases internal to a study are hard to detect. Bad data rarely self-identify[x]. A much safer and more persuasive course of action is for the expert

---

[u] See subsequent section – APPROPRIATE FACTS.

[v] Diagnoses should only be posed by competent, licensed medical professionals. And in any event, a life expectancy expert need not perform such examinations and instead may rely on appropriate medical reports, much like actuaries do not themselves examine prospective life insurance subscribers.

[w] Or, as mentioned, specialized reference manuals.[7]

[x] Although sometimes, internal inconsistencies are so crass and obvious as to belie serious methodological flaws. Such mistakes are usually caught by peer reviewers, but some journals – especially in the modern age of pay-to-publish – fail at this basic task. One should therefore examine not only the studies themselves, but their source (often a journal), both for reputation and track record.

to present a representative segment of the literature to demonstrate that the figures on which the opinion is built are not outlying or inappropriate values.

In the same vein, attention should be paid to the size of the studies on which the expert relies. Smaller studies are not per se incorrect, but the risk of spurious results is inversely proportional to the sample size. If the measured endpoint of a study is mortality, one will usually need a sample large enough to ensure enough measurable events (enough deaths). Although there is no strict threshold for validity, a study where the observed number of deaths is in the single digits should be examined with great care and reserve.

Similarly, the timeframe of studies is of great importance. Lengthy follow-ups are obviously costly, but studies that only capture a year of exposure are only of limited use. Mortality rates can progress over time, and often, the mortality of the first year following incidence is dramatically different from the long-term trend[y].

The selected studies should also be as relevant as feasible given the condition of interest. For example, if the patient suffers from diabetes to the point of neuropathy or nephropathy, it would definitely be improper under FRE 702 (d) to apply mortality rates from a study of all diabetics; the levels of mortality are simply not the same[z]. This speaks to a broader issue, which can be stated as follows: the best sources are the ones that, other things being equal, most closely relate to the condition. At the same time, one should also recognize that in some cases, the captured sample may be wider than desired. For example, in the case of coronary artery disease, a study may have as inclusion criterion an occlusion percentage of greater than 85%, when the case for which the expertise is sought has 95% occlusion. It is doubtful that one could find a study where the average occlusion is exactly the desired level. In such situations, the proper course of action would be to acknowledge the limitations and potential biases, but this would not wholly invalidate the analysis.

SUMMARY

Examining life expectancy opinions via the prism of evidentiary standards confers tangible benefits to the observer. This simple heuristic, although far from having perfect sensitivity, can highlight faults in the analysis, be they failure of qualification, methods, or facts. With this in mind, it can be useful for a witness tasked with producing a life expectancy opinion to keep in mind the commandments of the law as to the sufficiency of an opinion. Abiding by the requirements in a transparent fashion can not only ensure that the opinion will be deemed admissible, but also increase the likelihood that the opinion will be properly understood and appreciated by the finder of fact.

REFERENCES

1. Singer RB. How to prepare a life expectancy report for an attorney in a tort case. J Insur Med 2005;37:42–3.

2. Vachon PJ, Sestier F. Life expectancy determination. Phys Med Rehabil Clin N Am 2013;24(3):539–51.

---

[y] For instance, the mortality associated with spinal cord injury in the first year following injury is statistically different. In the case of stroke, the mortality is often dramatically higher in the first 30 days.

[z] Much like employing the average income level of all college graduates when the target is to estimate the expected income of a person with a doctorate, even though someone with a doctorate is necessarily a college graduate.

3. U.S. Federal Rules of evidence 702.
4. Ontario rules of civil Procedure, R.R.O. 1990, Reg. 194, r. 4.1.01, r. 53.03 as amended by O. Reg. 438/08, s. 8.
5. The human mortality database. Available at: http://www.mortality.org/hmd/USA/STATS/Mx_1x1.txt. Accessed August 2, 2018.
6. Graunt J. Natural and political observations mentioned in a following index, and made upon the bills of mortality 1662. London.
7. Brackenridge RDC, Croxson RS, Mackenzie BR. Medical selection of life risks. 5th edition.
8. Strauss DJ, Vachon PJ, Shavelle RM. Estimation of future mortality rates and life expectancy in chronic medical conditions. J Insur Med 2005;37:20–34.

Moving?

Make sure your subscription moves with you!

To notify us of your new address, find your **Clinics Account Number** (located on your mailing label above your name), and contact customer service at:

Email: journalscustomerservice-usa@elsevier.com

800-654-2452 (subscribers in the U.S. & Canada)
314-447-8871 (subscribers outside of the U.S. & Canada)

Fax number: 314-447-8029

Elsevier Health Sciences Division
Subscription Customer Service
3251 Riverport Lane
Maryland Heights, MO 63043

*To ensure uninterrupted delivery of your subscription, please notify us at least 4 weeks in advance of move.

Printed and bound by CPI Group (UK) Ltd, Croydon, CR0 4YY

03/10/2024

01040482-0001